Outline of Clinical Diagnosis in Cattle

Outline of Clinical Diagnosis in Cattle

A. H. Andrews, BVetMed, PhD, MRCVS
Senior Lecturer in Farm Animal Medicine,
Royal Veterinary College,
(University of London)

Wright
London Boston Singapore Sydney Toronto Wellington

Wright
is an imprint of Butterworth Scientific

 PART OF REED INTERNATIONAL P.L.C.

First published 1990

British Library Cataloguing in Publication Data
Andrews, A. H.
Outline of clinical diagnosis in cattle.
1. Livestock. Cattle. Diagnosis.
I. Title
636.2'0896075

ISBN 0–7236–0967–5

Library of Congress Cataloging in Publication Data
Andrews, A. H.
Outline of clinical diagnosis in cattle/A. H. Andrews.
p. cm.
ISBN 0–7236–0967–5
1. Cattle–Diseases–Diagnosis. I. Title.
[DNLM: 1. Cattle Diseases–diagnosis–outlines. SF 961 A565o]
SF961.A58 1990
636.2'0896075–dc20

Photoset by APS Ltd, Salisbury, Wiltshire.
Printed and bound by Hartnolls Ltd, Bodmin, Cornwall.

Preface

Any book covering differential diagnosis is bound to have some gaps and this is no exception. An attempt has been made to provide the most likely signs and then to list the conditions which result in these signs. Sometimes a generalized state is mentioned and in many of these there is a separate entry for that state which again will contain a list of possible causes. In a few instances where there are many causes of problems such as teat conditions, their more critical differentiation has been undertaken.

It is hoped the book will provide readers with a handy volume to keep by them when dealing with problematical cases. The list may then be used to jog the memory as to other possible diseases for consideration and investigation. None of the lists are comprehensive and should therefore be used only as a guide to likely problems.

As the book contains several new concepts, any observations or criticisms would be much appreciated.

Contents

Preface v

1 The art of diagnosis 1
2 Clinical examination 5
3 Alimentary system 59
4 Liver 97
5 Cardiovascular system 105
6 Respiratory system 115
7 Urinary system 131
8 Nervous system 139
9 Mammary gland 173
10 Skin 177
11 Musculoskeletal system 187
12 Genital system 195
13 Deaths 203
Index 207

1 The art of diagnosis

Diagnosis is the method of determining, to the best of one's ability from all the available information, why an animal is showing signs of abnormality in behaviour, or production, or a structural or functional change in all or part of its body. The art of diagnosis is of increasing importance to cattle clinicians today as they become more involved in tackling herd problems rather than dealing with individual animals. However, in all cases involving a group of animals, after reviewing the records and detailing the history, it becomes necessary to look at and assess individual animals. Clinical acumen becomes just as important in selecting the cattle to be examined as investigating those chosen. Mistakes in diagnosis can be expensive in terms of lost production, inappropriate treatment or preventive measures.

Whether dealing with a group or an individual animal, the main aim of any investigation is to determine why the animal is ill or, just as importantly these days, why certain production parameters are not being met. It is only by a careful and accurate examination, taking into account the history, signs and possibly laboratory tests, that a satisfactory diagnosis can be made. Only when this has been achieved can the correct therapy be instituted, a likely prognosis decided upon and adequate preventive measures suggested and instituted. Any diagnosis is one's opinion at a particular time, it should never be written in tablets of stone but should be fluid so that it can be altered or refined in the light of new evidence which becomes available as the disease progresses, further facts which are gleaned from the history, results of laboratory investigations or following response to treatment or preventive measures.

The only way a good clinician can work is by being completely familiar with the normal, healthy animal. Unfortunately this takes time and experience to acquire, and often considerable effort. This is because veterinary surgeons are called out to look at the abnormal rather than the healthy. It should also be remembered that an abnormality may be a compensatory reaction of cattle to their environment rather than the animals themselves being unhealthy. In such instances it is the conditions which are unhealthy and not the animals.

Normality is itself variable and although altered by extremes, it is also moderated by the management of the animals and the conditions under which they are kept. A simple example is that dairy cattle kept indoors in the winter will have a different consistency to their faeces if fed good quality hay or silage and either type will be correct for the diet given. Usually the differences are more subtle than this but should always be looked for on individual farms as well as in each form of accommodation or pasture used on a farm. A knowledge of animal behaviour is also necessary, as well as how it is influenced by other members of its group, the management undertaken and the conditions under which it is fed and kept. It is thus important never to be afraid to look at animals in the same situation which are considered to be healthy and then to assess and advise accordingly.

A good examination takes time and patience. It should not be hurried but, on the other hand, time should not be wasted. History can be collected or observations about the environment made while the general state of the group or individual is being assessed. If not undertaken satisfactorily then important points will be overlooked and these can be costly both to the farmer, in wrong advice and therapy being given, and to the veterinary surgeon, who will have his reputation reduced in the eyes of his client, or possibly even be required to provide some recompense for the oversight. Fortunately, or unfortunately, animal owners including farmers are becoming much more critical of the veterinary service they receive. They are also increasingly willing to undertake litigation where unsatisfactory outcomes have occurred.

When dealing with herd problems where the main sign is failure to reach production targets it may well be that the cattle are completely healthy but cannot perform better under the managemental, nutritional and environmental conditions in which they are kept. In consequence, following the initial examination of cattle and surroundings it will be necessary to perform a detailed analysis of management, nutrition and environment rather than of the animal itself. In such cases, 'treatment' is then an alteration of management in its broadest or a more specific sense.

2 Clinical examination

History taking
Examination of the animal or group
Identification
Clinical examination
General inspection
Specific appearance
Behaviour
Demeanour/temperament
Posture
Eating
Drinking
Dehydration
Defaecation
Urination
Respiration
Temperature
Pulse
Examination of the mucous membranes
- Colour
- Discharge

Examination of the lymph nodes
Examination of the environment
- Indoors
- Outdoors

The clinical examination can be divided into three parts, each of which is of great importance to the diagnosis:

1. History
2. Examination of the animal(s)
3. Examination of the environment(s).

While it is necessary to complete each phase, they are all interdependent. In consequence, although the natural order in which to proceed would perhaps be to follow that given above, in many cases it may be necessary as the animal is being examined to confirm or ask further about the history. The environmental findings may likewise require further history to be taken or another detailed look at the animal. Laboratory tests may also be influenced as much by the history and environmental findings as by the animal itself.

History

The first essential step is to obtain an adequate history. This is far easier said than done, because it is often easy for the clinician to be diverted by his own prejudices into certain lines of questioning, which can be aided or abetted by the person providing the history. It is thus just as important when taking a history to determine its value (Table 2.1) and this depends on assessing the person providing it. There are some stockmen so astute that often a completely accurate diagnosis can be obtained from listening to the description provided by him/her. However, this luxury is becoming less common as those attending the cattle have to deal with increasing numbers of animals and often a greater amount of other responsibilities. The time stockmen have to observe and assess becomes less and less so that often all that can be said is that the animal is 'not right' or the cow's milk yield has dropped (Tables 2.2, 2.3). In general terms, a better history is given by those closely associated with tending the animals than those who have a more managerial role. Often when dealing with major herd problems, however, it is the manager who is seen and it is difficult to have adequate time alone with the relevant stockman. In such a case the stockman may provide the answers which he feels the owner or manager wishes to hear. Worse still, the stockman may not be allowed to give his version of the problem because of continual interruption by his superior.

Table 2.1 Some factors to be considered when taking a history

Immediate
- Problem seen
- Other recent problems
- Other animals affected with similar signs
- Management changes prior to problem
- Recent changes in environment, e.g. weather, etc.
- Alterations in numbers of the group in which disease has occurred
- Introduction of new animals to the farm
- Treatments/nursing given
- Recent routine procedures (vaccination, disbudding, castration)

Past
- Management changes including:
  - housing changes
  - nutrition changes
  - labour changes
  - group composition changes
  - introduction of new animals to the farm
  - breeding policy
- Other animals previously ill or died
- Preventive measures undertaken

History-taking is a great art and is perhaps the more important part of the examination as it will lead to the rest of the diagnostic process. It is fraught with pitfalls. Often the clinician causes problems by asking leading questions which in themselves may help confirm his prejudices. There is also the problem that the person providing the information may exaggerate or misinform the clinician. Again this depends on assessing the reliability of the person providing the history. Misinformation can be deliberate, particularly if the person thinks the animal's problems are due in part to something which he/she has or has not done. In other cases information is proffered when in fact it would be more honest of the stockman to say he does not know.

The history obtained should be as accurate and complete as possible. However, it will very much depend on the human fallibilities of the person who does the interviewing as well as the interviewee. It should always be easier for a person who attends a farm regularly to obtain the relevant information quickly. This is because he should have a good idea of the aims of the farm, the routine management and feeding of the animals. It is thus easier for him to note changes which may be overlooked or forgotten by the stockman. There is, however,

Table 2.2 Milk yield: some causes of a sudden drop

A drop in milk yield is often the first indication of a disease process. There is usually some fall in all cases of pyrexia, pain or toxaemia. Less sudden falls most commonly occur as the result of a depression in appetite.

Abomasal torsion
Abomasal ulceration
Acidosis
Anthrax
Antibiotic inclusion in feed
Anorexia
Arsenic poisoning
Atypical interstitial pneumonia
Bacillary haemoglobinuria
Bovine malignant catarrh
Bovine viral diarrhoea
Change of ration
Colic
Contagious bovine pleuropneumonia
Displaced abomasum (right)
Endocarditis (periodic drop)
Fever
Foot-and-mouth disease
Foul in the foot
Gas gangrene
Indigestion, simple (usually slight drop)
Infectious bovine keratoconjunctivitis (few cases)
Infectious bovine rhinotracheitis
Lack of feed
Lack of water
Leptospirosis (acute)
Leptospira hardjo infection
Liver abscess necrobacillosis (acute)
Malignant oedema
Mouldy feed
Mouth lesions
Mucosal disease
Pain
Parasitic bronchitis
Pericarditis
Pulmonary abscess
Redwater fever
Rinderpest
Ruminal atony (usually slight drop)
Salmonellosis (acute enteritis)
Silage — poor quality or butyric
Tickborne fever
Tooth eruption
Toxaemia
Traumatic pericarditis
Traumatic reticulitis (severe)
Winter dysentery

Table 2.3 Milk yield: some causes of a gradual drop

Acetonaemia
Aflatoxicosis
Arthropathy
Caecal dilatation
Caecal torsion
Calcium deficiency
Contagious bovine pyelonephritis
Copper deficiency
Displaced abomasum (left-sided)
Fascioliasis
Hypomagnesaemia (subacute)
Johne's disease
Molybdenum poisoning
Osteomalacia
Phosphorus deficiency
Sodium chloride deficiency
Toxaemia (chronic)
Traumatic hepatitis
Traumatic splenitis
Tuberculosis

also the problem of familiarity breeding contempt and this can lead to some fundamental points being overlooked by the clinician. When dealing with a herd problem there is usually a tendency to take more time to obtain the history than when a single animal is involved. While this may seem correct in that the ramifications of the disease are more serious, correct history-taking in the individual should really take almost as long as for a group. One must also remember, of course, that in any disease outbreak there is always the first case and so the consequences of that individual case may be potentially just as serious as those in a herd problem.

Once a satisfactory history is obtained it can often be corroborated by the examination of the animal or its environment. Where this does not occur it is often useful to check the previous answers received by cross-questioning, i.e. using different questions which should provide answers similar to those already obtained. This is particularly the case when two or more people have been providing the information and there are disparities between their answers.

The history itself can be divided into *immediate history* and *past history* (*see* Table 2.1). Which is dealt with first is of less importance than ensuring both are obtained. Generally the immediate history is likely to be more forthcoming. This will often include how long the animal has been ill, any events leading up to the illness, whether it is a recurrence of a problem already seen in the herd or a condition in that particular animal, and the main reasons why the veterinary surgeon was called in. If undertaken thoroughly this should indicate whether the condition is acute or chronic and possibly the likelihood of it affecting others within the herd.

The duration of the problem often needs to be considered carefully because frequently these days the farmer will have treated the animal himself and it is only on the unsuccessful result of his own administrations that the clinician has been approached. This also means that careful investigation is necessary to determine what treatments and other changes of management and nursing have been undertaken since the animal was observed to be abnormal. It goes without saying that these changes are particularly important when it comes to examining the animal because the signs may well have been modified and the possible cause of the problem may have altered completely, if due to the environment or management.

The immediate history as suggested above does tend to merge into the past history. It is obviously important to know whether the condition has occurred previously in the animal under investigation, if any other animals have had similar problems and if so, whether they are of similar age and under similar management. Other illnesses over the last month or two in similar and other groups of animals should be determined. The introduction of new animals of any age should be found out as well as whether or not any management changes of environment, nutrition or labour have been instituted just prior to the problem occurring or perhaps in the last few months. As stated previously, it is to be hoped that the regular attendance of the veterinary surgeon will help considerably in knowing what these changes are and their likely influence on the herd or involvement in each particular farm setting. The history here should include any preventive measures which have been undertaken to reduce disease and which might be relevant to the problem under investigation.

Examination of the animal or group

Identification

This should first involve identification of the individual or group. This may seem academic but it is important to have some method of knowing which animal has been ill. At best it helps when producing an invoice, but it does enable recurrence of disease to be noted and, at worst, if things do go wrong, it allows accurate report production. All cattle over 2 weeks old should have some form of identification, even if it is only its herd and individual number which is required under the Tuberculosis Order 1964 and the Tuberculosis (Scotland) Order 1964.

When a group of animals is together it is often the case that other forms of identification are used including large ear tags, freeze branding, tail or neck bands. All these are helpful provided the form in which the number is recorded is noted, as any individual animal may have two or more different numbers present, depending on the reason for identification. There is a tendency, at present only small, to label animals electronically. While this is quite satisfactory for many purposes, it does require the animals' numbers to be read using some form of machine which may or may not be static. Such a system does not do away with the need for an easily visible method of identification for the clinician or the stockman who is working with the animals.

Where no easy way of identifying an ill animal is available, the use of a clip mark or a marker spray or stick can be helpful. Any recording should ideally also include breed of animal, its sex and approximate age.

Clinical examination

This obviously forms an essential part of the formation of any diagnosis. It also encompasses the collection of relevant samples and specimens for further investigation, usually in a laboratory. It is generally stated that clinical examination must always be thorough. This is true since in many cases more than one problem may be present in the same animal and unless a proper and systematic study is undertaken, one or other problem may be overlooked. However, often it is only necessary to undertake a rapid investigation of certain body systems of cattle to ascertain that they are normal. The examination can then be concentrated on those parts of the animal which indicate dysfunction or abnormality. Indeed, in some animals (but becoming rarer these days), the signs of illness presented suggest an uncomplicated disease. Usually inexperienced clinicians will require longer to undertake a clinical examination and will need to do this more thoroughly. This should never be thought a waste of time nor should it be discouraged because where misdiagnoses occur it is usually the fault of an experienced clinician not undertaking a thorough examination and jumping to the wrong conclusions.

A good clinical examination should lead to a tentative diagnosis. This may need further confirmation by re-questioning or considering new areas in the history or looking at the environment. In addition there should be an indication as to whether or not samples need to be taken. If sampling is necessary it should be possible to indicate which these should be. Ideally all diagnoses should be confirmed. Generally and practically, however, as laboratory diagnosis of disease adds to the cost, samples should only be taken where it is necessary to reach a diagnosis, to confirm the diagnosis for recording purposes, to ensure correct treatment or prevention is instituted, or where it may be necessary to produce reports which may be used by the clients in claims against third parties. Careful clinical examination will ensure all testing is kept to the minimum and is completely relevant to the particular case. Unfortunately there is sometimes a tendency to use laboratory tests as a means of diagnosis rather than an aid to it. It should always be remembered that clinical acumen is the veterinary surgeon's greatest asset because it allows an immediate answer to be given without extra cost to the client.

It is beyond the scope of this book to go into every detail of examination, however the general inspection of the animal will be discussed here. More specific factors involving the various body systems will be dealt with separately. Some clinicians favour moving from one area of the animal to another, i.e. from head to tail, taking in all aspects of the systems present in each region. This is effective but can sometimes lead to areas being omitted. Other clinicians work on a systematic approach, dealing with each system in turn. This does allow all areas to be examined in a methodical way but is time-consuming. Perhaps the best approach is to perform a rapid overall examination by region and then to concentrate on a systematic examination of those which suggest abnormality.

General inspection

This is the initial part of the examination and is of major importance (Table 2.4). Unfortunately it is often neglected or only performed in a cursory way. The inspection should be undertaken in an unhurried fashion and should involve as little disturbance to the animal as is possible. It can usually be carried

Table 2.4 General examination of the animal

General inspection

1. Identification (if possible at this stage)
2. General appearance
3. Physical condition
4. Specific appearance
   - skin condition
   - behaviour
   - demeanour
   - resting posture
   - standing posture
   - specific posture
   - gait
   - conformation
   - voice
   - eating
   - drinking
   - dehydration
   - defaecation
   - urination
   - respiration: rate, depth, dyspnoea, thoracic symmetry, rhythm, type, noises
   - temperature: rectal, skin
   - pulse: rate, rhythm, amplitude
   - visible mucous membranes: colour, discharges, swelling, haemorrhages
   - odours
   - lymph node examination

Regional examination

Coat and skin
Head
Neck
Thorax
Abdomen
Udder
Front limbs
Hind limbs

Systematic examination

Alimentary system
Respiratory system
Cardiovascular system
Genital system
Urinary system
Locomotory system
Nervous system

out at the same time as history is being obtained. The aim should be to observe both the animal and its surroundings. It should be performed looking over the door of a box or outside the rails of a pen. As cattle tend to be handled less and less then the inspection should be undertaken some feet from the animal. Ideally it should be viewed from both sides and at all angles to note any dysymmetry or localized problems.

The aim of a general inspection is firstly to identify abnormalities for more detailed investigation and secondly to observe signs which would otherwise be missed if the animal was disturbed or only viewed at close proximity. The general

Table 2.5 Some causes of poor growth

Abomasal ulceration
Arsenic poisoning (chronic)
Bullying
Calcium deficiency
Carbohydrate deficiency
Chronic infections
Chronic localized peritonitis
Chronic suppurative pneumonia
Cobalt deficiency
Coccidiosis
Copper deficiency
Cuffing pneumonia
Eisenmenger's syndrome
Endocarditis
Fascioliasis
Fluorosis (chronic)
Malnutrition
Mannosidosis
Mucosal disease
Pantothenic acid deficiency (calves)
Parasitic bronchitis
Parasitic gastroenteritis
Phosphorus deficiency
Potassium deficiency
Protein deficiency
Pyridoxine deficiency (calves)
Riboflavin deficiency (calves)
Salmonellosis
Selenium/vitamin E deficiency
Suppurative arthritis
Suppurative pneumonia, chronic
Tetralogy of Fallot
Undernutrition
Urachus infection
Vitamin A deficiency
Water deprivation

inspection should be followed in a routine way, but the order in which it is undertaken is a matter for personal preference.

General appearance

The appearance of the animal may be normal or it may be large or small for its age. Its general bone structure may be fine or thick and this is particularly noticeable in the limbs. The skeletal characteristics are obviously partly dependent on the breed, but they are also affected by the animal's own genetics, environment and management.

Specific appearance

The limbs may show signs of deformity. Various swellings may be apparent on different parts of the body or there may be asymmetry.

Skin The appearance of the animal's coat should be noted as being healthy or showing signs of neglect or debility (Table 2.8).

Table 2.6 Some causes of poor condition

Abomasal dilatation (chronic – gradual loss)
Abomasal impaction (later stages)
Acetonaemia
Actinobacillosis
Actinomycosis
Alimentary neoplasia (loss of condition)
Bovine spongiform encephalopathy
Bracken poisoning
Cobalt deficiency
Coccidiosis
Congestive heart failure
Contagious bovine pleuropneumonia (chronic)
Copper deficiency
Diaphragmatic hernia (over several weeks)
Enzootic bovine leukosis
Erysipelas infection
Fascioliasis
Foot-and-mouth disease
Hypomagnesaemia (chronic loss)
Iron deficiency (calves)
Lice infestation
Mucosal disease
Osteomalacia
Oxalate poisoning (chronic)
Parasitic bronchitis
Parasitic gastroenteritis
Sodium chloride poisoning
Sodium deficiency
Tuberculosis (*Mycobacterium tuberculosis*)
Zinc deficiency

Table 2.7 Some causes of emaciation

Actinobacillosis (neglected)
Actinomycosis
Amyloidosis
Bovine spongiform encephalopathy
Carbon tetrachloride poisoning (chronic)
Chlorinated naphthalene poisoning
Cobalt deficiency
Contagious pyelonephritis
Copper deficiency
Degenerative joint disease
Enzootic bovine leukosis
Fascioliasis
Haemonchosis
Johne's disease
Liver abscess necrobacillosis (acute)
Malnutrition
Mercury poisoning (chronic)
Molybdenum poisoning
Oesophagostomiasis
Ostertagiasis Type II
Parasitic gastroenteritis
Pharyngeal obstruction
Pulmonary abscess
Pyrexia/pruritus/haemorrhagic syndrome
Redwater fever
Sarcosporidiosis
Sporadic bovine leukosis
Starvation
Toxaemia (chronic)
Tuberculosis (*Mycobacterium bovis*)
Upper alimentary squamous cell carcinoma
Water deprivation

Table 2.8 Hair: rough, harsh, staring

Arsenic poisoning
Chronic diarrhoea
Cobalt deficiency
Copper deficiency
Fascioliasis
Manganese deficiency
Molybdenum poisoning
Pantothenic acid deficiency
Parasitic gastroenteritis
Phosphorus deficiency
Pyridoxine deficiency
Rinderpest
Tapeworm infestation
Tuberculosis (*Mycobacterium bovis* – some cases)

Condition

The general body condition of the animal in terms of its degree of thinness or fatness should be assessed as well as its size in relation to breed, age and sex (Table 2.5). The animal may show loss of weight (Table 2.6) and, if extreme, it is emaciated (Table 2.7). A gradual slow loss of condition can occur and is generally known as cachexia. Often the assessment of condition score is helpful.

Behaviour

The animal may show signs of abnormal behaviour, being separated from the rest of the herd.

Demeanour/temperament

This varies with age and sex. However, the animal may seem dull (Table 2.9) or excessively alert. It may also show depressed or exaggerated responses to stimuli such as light, sound, movement, etc. (Tables 2.10 and 2.11). The animal may show dullness or apathy which in a more severe form leads to sleepiness (Table 2.12) or coma (Table 2.13). In the case of

Table 2.9 Some causes of mild dullness

Arsenic poisoning
Cerebral anoxia (chronic)
Coenurosis
Fascioliasis
Fever
Gid
Haemorrhage
Heat stroke
Hyperthermia
Hypomagnesaemia (chronic)
Indigestion (simple)
Lead poisoning
Listeria infection (meningoencephalitis)
Milk allergy
Parasitic gastroenteritis
Pulmonary abscess
Ruminal atony
Selenium/vitamin E deficiency
Selenium poisoning (chronic)
Septicaemia
Shock

Table 2.10 Some causes of mild depression

Acetonaemia
Diphtheria – calf (stomatitis)
Encephalitis
Hydrocyanic acid poisoning (acute)
Indigestion (simple)
Listeria infection (septicaemia)
Lupinosis
Mercury poisoning (chronic)
Nephrosis
Osteomyelitis
Pneumonia
Ruminal atony
Sporadic bovine leukosis

increased response this can be seen as a mildly anxious animal with a greater alertness but normal movements. This may progress to restlessness which may be more or less continuous and can lead to mania and aggression (Table 2.14) when there may be compulsive movements undertaken with vigour. Frenzy is followed by wild, uncontrollable action.

Resting posture

The animal may be recumbent which, although a normal position, may be because it is unable to rise. It may also show other abnormalities in the positioning of its head or neck or general weakness (Table 2.15). Recumbency which is lateral rather than sternal is abnormal in most instances (Table 2.16).

Standing posture

Abnormalities of posture are variable indicating the nature of the problem. There may be alteration in the positioning of the limbs which may show rigidity. Most of these postural changes suggest abnormalities in the musculoskeletal or nervous systems. However, some alterations are not due to disease but can be the result of weakness or tiredness.

Specific posture

Some cattle may show elevation of the tail, rigidity of the ears, etc.

Table 2.11 Some causes of profound depression

Anthrax
Blackleg
Bovine malignant catarrh
Bovine viral diarrhoea
Brain abscess
Carbon tetrachloride poisoning
Circulation failure, peripheral
Colisepticaemia (calves)
Congestive heart failure
Contagious bovine pleuropneumonia
Diphtheria (laryngeal)
Displaced abomasum (right-sided)
Electrocution
Encephalitis
Enteric toxaemia (*Escherichia coli*, calves)
Foot-and-mouth disease
Gas gangrene
Haemophilus somnus infection
Hepatitis
Hydrocephalus
Infectious bovine rhinotracheitis (calf encephalitis)
Intestinal obstruction, acute
Lightning strike
Liver abscess necrobacillosis (acute)
Malignant oedema
Mucosal disease
Pasteurellosis (pneumonic)
Peritonitis (acute diffuse)
Pharyngeal phlegmon
Photosensitization (severe)
Pleurisy
Redwater fever
Salmonellosis (septicaemia – calves)
Sulphur poisoning
Toxaemia
Traumatic pericarditis
Traumatic reticulitis (with acute diffuse peritonitis)

Table 2.12 Some causes of sleepiness (somnolence)

Carbon tetrachloride poisoning
Ergot poisoning (acute)
Haemophilus somnus infection
Hepatitis (some cases)
Listeria infection (meningoencephalitis)
Parturient paresis
Sodium chlorate poisoning
Zinc poisoning (severe)

Table 2.13 Some causes of coma

Some causes of coma
Arsenic poisoning
Bladder rupture
Ergot poisoning (acute)
Fat cow syndrome (beef, late signs dairy)
Haemorrhage, acute (some)
Heat stroke
Hepatitis (some cases)
Hyperthermia
Hypothermia
Lead poisoning
Meningitis (later signs)
Parturient paresis
Phosphorus poisoning
Shock (severe)
Transit tetany

Table 2.14 Some causes of aggressive behaviour

Some causes of aggressive behaviour
Anabolic steroid implants/usage (a few)
Bovine spongiform encephalopathy
Bulls
Cystic ovaries
Fat cow syndrome
Hepatitis (some)
Mannosidosis
Maternal (cow with calf)
Rabies
Testosterone implants
Virilism in cow

Gait

When the animal is allowed to walk unrestricted it may show abnormalities. Points which need to be considered include:

1. rate
2. force
3. range, and
4. direction of movement.

Ideally this should be assessed when the animal is free to move naturally. The animal should move towards, away from and past the observer. It may be quick or slow or reluctant (Table 2.17) in its movements. It may show a shortened stride or a

Table 2.15 Some causes of weakness

Weakness can be the result of lack of feed intake, muscle weakness or it can be due to nervous or circulatory problems.

Carbon tetrachloride poisoning
Cerebral anoxia (chronic)
Choline deficiency (calves)
Circulation failure, peripheral
Cobalt deficiency
Colienteritis (calves)
Colisepticaemia (calves)
Displaced abomasum (right-sided)
Endocarditis
Enteric toxaemia (*Escherichia coli* calves)
Enzootic bovine leukosis
Enzootic haematuria
Fascioliasis (chronic)
Fat cow syndrome
Fever
Gas gangrene
Haemorrhage
Haemophilus somnus infection
Hepatitis (some cases)
Hormone weedkiller poisoning (calves)
Johne's disease
Kale poisoning
Listeria infection (septicaemia)
Liver abscess necrobacillosis (acute)
Malignant catarrh
Mercury poisoning (chronic)
Myopathy
Osteomalacia
Parasitic gastroenteritis
Peritonitis, acute diffuse (with toxaemia)
Phosphorus poisoning
Photosensitization (severe)
Post-parturient haemoglobinuria
Ragwort poisoning
Redwater fever
Selenium/vitamin E deficiency (subacute)
Septicaemia
Shock
Sodium chlorate poisoning (chronic)
Sporadic bovine leukosis (generalized)
Thiamine deficiency
Toxaemia
Vagal indigestion (ruminal atony – late stages)
Vitamin A deficiency
Vitamin B_{12} deficiency (calves)
Water intoxication

Table 2.16 Some causes of recumbency

Abomasal impaction (later stages)
Abomasal torsion
Acidosis
Anaemia
Arsenic poisoning
Arthropathy (prolonged periods)
Babesiosis
Botulism (lateral)
Bovine spongiform encephalopathy
Cereal overeating
Cerebral anoxia (acute)
Choline deficiency (calves)
Downer cow
Endocarditis
Enzootic haematuria
Erysipelas arthritis
Fat cow syndrome
Foot-and-mouth disease
Haemophilus somnus infection
Haemorrhage
Hepatitis (some cases)
Hormone weedkiller poisoning
Hydrocyanic acid poisoning
Hypomagnesaemia (lateral)
Inherited hypermotility of gut
Inherited neuraxial oedema
Inherited reduced phalagy
Listeria infection (meningoencephalitis)
Louping ill
Osteomalacia
Oxalate poisoning (acute)
Parturient paresis (sternal – mid stages; lateral – late stages)
Post-parturient haemoglobinuria
Peritonitis, acute diffuse (with toxaemia)
Phosphorus deficiency (particularly late pregnancy)
Rickets
Ruminal tympany
Selenium/vitamin E deficiency (acute – lateral; subacute – sternal)
Shock
Tetanus
Transit tetany
Traumatic pericarditis (later stages)
Traumatic reticulitis (some cases)
Vagal indigestion (ruminal atony – late stages)

stilted gait. Occasionally there may be shuffling or exaggerated movements. There may be stiffness or lameness. In other cases the animal will show excessive abduction or adduction of the limbs, or there may be swinging of the hindlimbs, staggering or swaying.

Table 2.17 Some causes of reluctance to move

Acetonaemia
Arsenic poisoning
Bacillary haemoglobinuria
Fog fever
Hepatitis
Hydrocephalus
Hypertrophic pulmonary osteoarthropathy
Laminitis
Lameness
Lead poisoning
Manganese deficiency
Molybdenum poisoning
Parturient paresis (early stages)
Pericarditis
Peritonitis, acute diffuse
Pleurisy
Renal calculi (pelvic blockage)
Rickets
Traumatic pericarditis
Traumatic reticulitis
Tuberculosis (*Mycobacterium bovis*)

Conformation

This involves checking that the animal shows symmetry and that a particular part of the body is not disproportionate to the rest.

Voice

Changes in the voice are uncommon in cattle. Occasionally, however, there is persistent lowing. Less likely are soundless bellowing or yawning.

Eating

The animal may show difficulty in prehension, mastication or swallowing or be reluctant to eat. This can result in reduced appetite (Table 2.18) or complete loss of appetite – anorexia (Table 2.19). There can be cuds present in the mouth or dropped around the box or pen. The presence or absence of food in the pen can give an indication as to the animal's appetite or perhaps frequency of feeding. Prehension may be difficult with, in some cases, inability to reach the feed or, in other cases, problems of transfer to the mouth. Chewing may result in signs of

Table 2.18 Some causes of reduced appetite

Abomasitis (acute)
Abomasitis (chronic)
Acetonaemia
Blue tongue
Calcium deficiency
Cobalt deficiency
Copper deficiency
Displaced abomasum (left-sided)
Displaced abomasum (right-sided)
Enzootic bovine leukosis
Enzootic pneumonia (calves)
Hyperaemia (subacute)
Indigestion, simple
Infections
Infectious bovine keratoconjunctivitis
Iron deficiency
Lead poisoning (subacute)
Molybdenosis
Osteomyelitis
Oxalate poisoning (chronic)
Parturient paresis
Post-parturient haemoglobinuria
Pyrexia
Ruminal atony
Sodium chloride poisoning (chronic)
Vagal indigestion (ruminal atony)
Vagal indigestion (signs for prolonged period)
Vitamin A deficiency
Vitamin D deficiency

discomfort and there may be excessive salivation as evidenced by drooling of saliva or wetness around the mouth.

Drinking

The animal may show signs of excessive thirst and position itself over the drinking trough. It may show a reluctance or difficulty in drinking.

Dehydration

Dehydration reaches variable degrees (Table 2.20). There are two main causes of dehydration: lack of water intake is usually due to water deprivation or possibly a lack of thirst as occurs in conditions such as toxaemia, or a physical problem preventing drinking (e.g. pharyngeal paralysis, oesophageal obstruction).

Table 2.19 Some causes of anorexia (complete loss of appetite)

Abomasal dilatation
Abomasal impaction (complete)
Abomasal torsion
Abomasal ulceration
Abomasitis (acute)
Acidosis (often complete)
Alimentary neoplasia
Anthrax
Arsenic poisoning
Bacillary haemoglobinuria
Blackleg
Botulism
Bovine malignant catarrh
Bovine viral diarrhoea
Bronchitis
Caecal dilatation
Caecal torsion
Carbon tetrachloride poisoning
Cereal engorgement (often complete)
Choline deficiency (calves)
Circulation failure, peripheral
Colienteritis (calves)
Colisepticaemia (calves)
Contagious bovine pleuropneumonia
Copper poisoning
Diphtheria (laryngeal)
Diphtheria (stomatitis) (calf)
Displaced abomasum (left)
Displaced abomasum (right)
Encephalitis
Enteric toxaemia (calves)
Fat cow syndrome
Fascioliasis
Fodder beet poisoning
Foot-and-mouth disease
Gas gangrene
Indigestion (simple)
Infections (severe)
Infectious bovine rhinotracheitis
Hepatitis
Hormone weedkiller poisoning
Laryngitis
Leptospira hardjo infection
Leptospirosis (acute)
Liver abscess (necrobacillosis – acute, chronic)
Lupinosis
Malignant oedema
Mangel poisoning
Mercury poisoning (acute, chronic)
Mucosal disease
Oesophagostomiasis

Table 2.19 continued

Omasal atony (acute)
Peritonitis (acute diffuse) (complete)
Pharyngeal phlegmon
Pharyngitis
Pleurisy
Pneumonia
Pulmonary abscess
Pyrexia
Pyridoxine deficiency (calves)
Rabies
Redwater fever
Riboflavin deficiency
Rinderpest
Ruminal atony
Salmonellosis (acute enteritis)
Sarcosporidiosis
Septicaemia
Sodium chloride poisoning
Stomatitis
Sugar beet poisoning
Thiamine deficiency
Toxaemia
Tracheitis
Transit tetany
Traumatic pericarditis (complete)
Traumatic reticulitis (complete)
Vagal indigestion (pyloric obstruction)
Vitamin A deficiency
Vitamin B_{12} deficiency (calf)

Table 2.20 Signs of dehydration in calves

Bodyweight loss (%)	*Signs*	*PCV* (%)
4–6	Normal	40
6–8	Dry muzzle, mouth and mucous membranes, sunken eyes, decreased skin elasticity. Tenting 2–4 s	50
8–10	Cold legs and oral cavity, often recumbent. Tenting 6–10 s	55
10–12	Comatosed and in shock. Tenting 20–45 s	60
Over 12	Death	

PCV: packed cell volume

The main cause of dehydration is, however, an excessive loss of fluid as in diarrhoea, intestinal or abomasal obstruction, etc. (Table 2.21).

Defaecation

This may be difficult, as with constipation or painful abdominal conditions. It can also be relatively involuntary when diarrhoea is present.

Urination

The act of micturition may appear to be difficult and result in pain. Micturition can be more frequent than normal and occasionally there may be incontinence.

Table 2.21 Some causes of dehydration

Abomasal dilatation (acute)
Abomasal impaction
Abomasal ulceration with perforation
Abomasitis (acute)
Acidosis
Bovine viral diarrhoea (acute)
Brewers' grain poisoning
Caecal dilatation (mild)
Caecal torsion (mild)
Cereal overload
Diarrhoea
Displaced abomasum (right-sided)
Enteritis
Heat stroke
Hyperthermia
Johne's disease
Lack of thirst
Mercury poisoning
Mucosal disease
Oesophageal obstruction
Parasitic gastroenteritis
Pharyngeal paralysis
Post-parturient haemoglobinuria
Rinderpest
Shock
Sodium chloride poisoning (chronic)
Thiamine deficiency (calves)
Toxaemia
Viral diarrhoea (calves)

Respiration

The animal's respirations need to be assessed before entering the box or pen and thereby disturbing the animal. The rate, depth, rhythm and character of the movements are all assessed.

Respiratory rate

Normal respiratory rate for cattle = 10–30/min; abnormal >40/min (Tables 2.22, 2.23). The rate can be counted by watching the rise and fall of the thoracic rib cage, by observing the nostril movements, by auscultation of the trachea or thorax, or by palpation of the nasal air movements. As with other parameters, the respiratory rate varies in normal animals. It tends to be higher (tachypnoea, polypnoea) in younger animals as well as following exercise, exertion or excitement. It is considered to be abnormal when about 40/min, which may be a result of the animal's environment. It tends to be high if the temperature or relative humidity are high. Cattle used to being outside in cold temperatures may show mouth breathing and panting with the respiratory rate at least six times the previous level within only two hours after housing. A rise is also seen when cattle have a fever or respiratory disease such as pneumonia, pleurisy, obstruction of the respiratory passages, cardiac disease and anoxia.

Decreased rate is known as oligpnoea and is rare, although it may occur when environmental conditions are cold. It can occur when there are space-occupying lesions affecting the respiratory

Table 2.22 Some causes of increase in respiration

Abomasal impaction
Circulation failure, peripheral
Congestive heart failure (left)
Contagious bovine pleuropneumonia
Kale poisoning
Pain
Peritonitis, acute diffuse
Pulmonary congestion
Pulmonary emphysema
Pulmonary oedema
Pyrexia
Traumatic pericarditis
Traumatic reticulitis
Tuberculosis (*Mycobacterium avium*)
Tuberculosis (*Mycobacterium bovis*)

Table 2.23 Some causes of rapid respiration

Acidosis
Anthrax
Arsenic poisoning
Aspiration pneumonia
Atypical interstitial pneumonia
Bovine farmer's lung
Bovine viral diarrhoea
Cereal overload
Choline deficiency (calves)
Contagious bovine pleuropneumonia
Crude oil poisoning
Dinitrophenol poisoning
Fat cow syndrome (beef)
Fog fever
Haemophilus somnus infection
Heat stroke
Hyperthermia
Hypomagnesaemia
Infectious bovine rhinotracheitis
Lungworm infestation
Mercury poisoning
Milk allergy
Mucosal disease
Nitrate/nitrite poisoning
Pain
Pasteurellosis (pneumonic)
Pericarditis
Pleurisy
Pneumonia
Pulmonary emphysema
Pyrexia
Redwater fever
Ruminal tympany (up to 60)
Salmonellosis (acute enteritis)
Shock
Thrombosis of vena cava
Tickborne fever

centre, in uraemia and stenosis of the upper respiratory tract. Complete cessation of breathing is known as apnoea.

Depth

The depth is determined by noting the movement of the ribs and abdominal muscles. It can be normal, which means that the respirations can be observed but have to be consciously looked for. The amplitude can be increased (hyperpnoea) (Table 2.24) or decreased (hypopnoea) (Table 2.25). In hyperpnoea the movements of both the thorax and abdomen (Table 2.26) are

Table 2.24 Respiration: some causes of increased depth, hyperpnoea

Anthrax
Bovine farmer's lung
Chronic bovine pleuropneumonia
Congestive heart failure (left)
Dinitrophenol poisoning
Fever
Haemorrhage
Kale poisoning
Lungworm infestation (subacute)
Pulmonary congestion
Pulmonary emphysema
Pulmonary oedema
Septicaemia
Thrombosis of vena cava
Tuberculosis (*Mycobacterium avium*)
Tuberculosis (*Mycobacterium bovis*)

Table 2.25 Some causes of shallow respiration

Acidosis
Cereal overload
Circulation failure, peripheral
Contagious bovine pleuropneumonia
Haemophilus somnus infection
Heat stroke
Hyperthermia
Infectious bovine rhinotracheitis
Lungworm infestation (acute)
Pasteurellosis (pneumonic)
Pericarditis
Pleurisy
Pneumonia
Salmonellosis (acute enteritis)
Shock

Table 2.26 Some causes of abdominal respiration

Parasitic bronchitis
Pericarditis
Pharyngeal obstruction
Pleurisy
Pneumonia
Pulmonary congestion
Pulmonary oedema
Traumatic pericarditis

clearly visible and this is normally seen with exercise. Very deep respirations are considered to be laboured and are known as dyspnoea.

Dyspnoea (Table 2.27)
Dyspnoea results in other respiratory signs such as dilated nostrils, outstretched head and neck, mouth breathing, abduction of the elbows and a marked increase in the movement of the thoracic and abdominal walls. Respiratory sounds tend to be marked, including grunting.

Dyspnoea varies in degree from slight to moderate or severe. If an animal with dyspnoea is exercised or excited, the more severe the dyspnoea the longer the animal will take to recover. Inspiratory dyspnoea occurs where there is obstruction to the entry of air into the lungs and so transfer of oxygen to the blood is reduced. This happens in bronchopneumonia, pulmonary oedema, pulmonary congestion, pleurisy, hydrocyanide poisoning, methaemoglobin formation, stenosis of the air passages, diaphragmatic rupture, pulmonary emphysema. Expiratory dyspnoea occurs when air cannot leave the lungs properly, and is seen as protracted expiration with the formation of a pleuritic ridge.

Thoracic symmetry
Asymmetrical respiration can occur where there is widespread disease involving only one lung. This results in the healthy side moving to a normal or increased extent.

Rhythm
There are three phases to each normal respiratory cycle: inspiration, expiration and a pause. Usually the three phases are roughly equal in time, although expiration often takes slightly longer than inspiration. The duration of the pause is dependent on whether the animal is resting and relaxed or has recently been exercised or excited. During inspiration the costal arch moves outwards and slightly forwards. Inspiration involves the active movement of the diaphragm, abdominal and thoracic muscles initiated by the respiratory reflex. Thus in all cattle there is some abdominal movement on respiration. Expiration results in the costal arch moving inwards and slightly backwards. This action is mainly passive and is the result of the lungs contracting with collapse of the thoracic wall.

Prolongation of the inspiratory phase can be the result of obstruction in the upper respiratory tract. Increased duration of

Table 2.27 Some causes of dyspnoea

Abomasal dilatation (acute)
Actinomycosis (maxillary involvement)
Anaphylaxis
Anthrax
Aspergillosis pneumonia (calf)
Atypical interstitial pneumonia
Aujeszky's disease
Bacillary haemoglobinuria (terminally)
Bovine malignant catarrh
Bracken poisoning (calves)
Bronchitis
Candida spp. pneumonia
Chlorinated hydrocarbon poisoning
Choline deficiency
Congestive heart failure
Contagious bovine pleuropneumonia
Diphtheria (laryngeal)
Emphysema
Enzootic bovine leukosis (cardiac/respiratory form)
Fluorosis (acute)
Fog fever
Foot-and-mouth disease (cardiac form)
Haemophilus somnus infection
Haemothorax
Heart failure (acute)
Hydrocyanic acid poisoning
Hydrothorax
Hypersensitivity reaction
Infectious bovine rhinotracheitis
Kale poisoning
Laryngitis (inspiratory)
Leptospirosis (acute)
Listeria infection (septicaemia – calves)
Lungworm infestation
Lupin poisoning
Metaldehyde deficiency
Milk allergy
Monochloroacetate poisoning
Myocardial weakness
Nitrate/nitrite poisoning
Parasitic bronchitis
Pasteurellosis, pneumonic (severe)
Pharyngeal obstruction
Pharyngeal phlegmon
Photosensitization (nasal obstruction)
Pneumonia
Pneumothorax
Pulmonary congestion
Pulmonary emphysema (acute)
Pulmonary emphysema (chronic)
Pulmonary neoplasia

Table 2.27 continued
Pulmonary oedema
Rickets
Rinderpest
Ruminal tympany
Selenium/vitamin E deficiency (acute, subacute)
Sodium chlorate poisoning
Summer snuffles
Toxoplasmosis
Tracheitis (inspiratory)
Traumatic pericarditis
Tuberculosis (*Mycobacterium bovis*)
Urea poisoning
Yew poisoning

---

the expiratory phase is due to the inability of the lungs to collapse as occurs in emphysema. When respiratory disease occurs the pause is often lost and so the cycle becomes two-phase consisting only of inspiration and expiration.

Irregular respiration occurs commonly. It can be quite normal when breathing is interrupted when animals are distracted or investigating and sniffing. Dropped respirations can also occur. Cheyne-Stokes respiration is where the abnormal breathing involves periods of apnoea lasting 15–30 s, followed by a gradual increase in amplitude, then a gradual decrease which again leads into a period of apnoea. This type of respiration is usually seen in advanced cases of renal or cardiac disease. Biot's respiration is seen as periods of relatively shallow, rapid breathing followed by periods of apnoea. The duration of the polypnoea and respiratory movement vary in length. This type of respiration can occur in meningitis, particularly when the medulla oblongata is involved. Periodic breathing with periods of apnoea followed by short bouts of hyperventilation are seen in electrolyte and acid–base disturbances.

Type

This involves observing how the respiratory movements involve the thorax and abdomen. In normal cattle, movement of both the thorax and abdomen would occur but the movement is predominantly abdominal. There can be a marked exaggeration of the abdominal movement in painful thoracic conditions such as acute pleurisy or in intercostal muscle paralysis or emphysema. Thoracic immobility results in an expanded thorax and a pleuritic ridge. Predominantly thoracic breathing occurs when there are painful conditions in the abdomen such as peritonitis or when the action of the diaphragm is impaired due to paralysis, rupture or accumulation of gas or fluid in the abdomen as in ruminal tympany or hydrops amnii.

Noises

Various respiratory noises or stridors can be heard. These include sneezing when there is irritation of the nasal passages. More commonly there is coughing due to irritation of the pharynx, trachea or bronchi. Snoring or stertor (Table 2.28) is the result of pharyngeal obstruction. Wheezing can result from stenosis of the nasal passages.

Temperature

The temperature of cattle is usually measured *per rectum* with a clinical thermometer, usually the mercury type, although some are now electronic. Where it is impossible to obtain a rectal reading the thermometer can be inserted *per vaginam*. Maintenance of the body temperature is undertaken by balancing the amount of heat produced with that lost from the body. Loss of heat is by radiation, conduction, convection and evaporation. Heat is produced by the metabolism of the animal and muscular activity. Animals do not have a constant normal temperature. Large amounts of heat are lost when cattle lie on cold or wet ground or damp bedding. Animals which are fat tend to sweat but more especially lose heat by increasing their respiratory rate, which may lead to panting.

Table 2.28 Some causes of stertorous (snoring) respiration

Actinobacillosis
Botulism (some cases)
Bovine malignant catarrh
Bronchitis
Enlarged soft palate
Enlarged retropharyngeal lymph nodes
Enzootic bovine leukosis (respiratory form)
Kale poisoning
Laryngitis
Pharyngeal obstruction
Pharyngeal paralysis
Soft palate enlargement
Sporadic bovine leukosis
Summer snuffles
Tracheitis
Tuberculosis (*Mycobacterium bovis*)

Rectal temperature is capable of considerable variation and in the individual this can be around 1°C (2°F) due to diurnal variation from a high in the late afternoon to a low in the early morning. The temperature tends to increase when the cow or heifer is in oestrus, and it also rises by about 0.5°C (1°F) in late pregnancy. At the time of parturition, i.e. the last 24–48 h, there is a fall of about 0.5°C (1°F) and this is also seen just before the start of oestrus and at ovulation.

Temperature rises (hyperthermia) for various reasons. It can be because animals are placed in a warm environment or that those accustomed to low temperatures are brought indoors. In fact the temperature can reach abnormal proportions within two to four hours of housing. A rise in temperature can be the onset of pyrexia or fever and is accompanied by toxaemia; this occurs in most viral, bacterial and protozoal conditions. Other cases can be due to increased exercise, or abnormal muscular activity. Pain can also result in hyperthermia.

Reduction in temperature, or hypothermia (Table 2.29), can be the result of exposure to a cold environment or due to the inability of an animal to adapt to its environment. In other cases it can result from shock, toxaemia, circulatory collapse, metabolic disease or hypothyroidism. Animals close to death also tend to have lowered rectal temperatures. The temperature of younger animals tends to be higher than in those which are older.

	Normal	*Range*
Cattle	38.6°C (101.5°F)	38.0–39.5°C (100.4–103.1°F)
Calves	38.9°C (102.0°F)	38.6–39.7°C (101.5–103.5°F)

Fever (pyrexia)

This is a complex condition, involving both toxaemia (Table 2.30) and hyperthermia, which is usually the result of infectious disease. The stages of fever are traditionally divided into three and usually involve a sudden rise, a peak and then a fall which can result in the temperature being lower than before. The three stages are:

1. The onset – stage of increasing temperature. At this stage the internal body temperature is rising but there is a reduction in superficial circulation. Thus the animal feels cold and so shivers. This stage is called *stadium incrementi*.
2. Acme – which is the period of maximum temperature (*fastigium*).

Table 2.29 Some causes of subnormal temperature

Abomasal impaction
Abomasal torsion
Cereal engorgement
Circulation failure, peripheral
Colienteritis (calves)
Diarrhoea
Enteric toxaemia (*Escherichia coli* calves)
Haemorrhages
Hypothermia
Nephrosis
Nitrate/nitrite poisoning
Parturient paresis
Peritonitis, acute diffuse (with toxaemia)
Shock
Sodium chlorate poisoning
Toxaemia

Table 2.30 Some causes of toxaemia

Toxaemia is the result of toxin presence which can be caused by the breakdown of cells or from bacteria.

Aspiration pneumonia
Bronchitis
Colonic torsion
Crude oil poisoning
Dermatitis (extensive)
Embolic nephritis
Enteritis
Enzootic pneumonia (calves)
Intestinal obstruction
Laryngitis
Mastitis
Meningitis
Metritis
Myositis
Peritonitis, acute diffuse
Peritonitis, chronic
Pleurisy
Pneumonia
Tracheitis

3. Defervescence – the period of falling temperature (*stadium decrementi*).

The third stage can take place slowly or quickly. If there is a rapid fall this is known as a crisis but if the fall is more gradual it is called lysis. A rise in temperature but still within the normal range is described as sub-febrile. Fever can be categorized as being mild – 1°C (2°F) above normal (Table 2.31), moderately severe – 1.7–2.2°C (3–4°F) (Table 2.32) and severe – 2.8–3.3°C (5–6°F) above the usual level (Table 2.33).

Fever can be described by its type:

1. Simple or typical fever. This follows the three stages previously described with the temperature remaining high

Table 2.31 Some causes of mild pyrexia: 39.7–40.3°C (103.5–104.5°F)

Anaphylaxis
Bacillary haemoglobinuria
Brain abscess (some cases)
Bronchitis
Candida spp. pneumonia
Coccidiosis (mild)
Contagious bovine pleuropneumonia
Contagious bovine pyelonephritis
Crude oil poisoning
Cuffing pneumonia (calves)
Dinitrophenol poisoning
Diphtheria, calf (stomatitis)
Displaced abomasum (some)
Encephalitis
Endocarditis (fluctuating)
Enzootic bovine leukosis (some)
Fever
Foul in the foot (some)
Infectious bovine keratoconjunctivitis (few cases)
Laryngitis
Listeria infection (abortion, meningoencephalitis – early)
Osteomyelitis
Parasitic gastroenteritis
Pericarditis
Peritonitis, acute diffuse
Pleurisy
Pneumonia
Post-parturient haemoglobinuria
Sarcosporidiosis
Septicaemia
Septic arthritis
Streptococcal meningitis (calves)
Sporadic bovine leukosis (some cases)
Tetanus
Toxaemia
Toxoplasmosis
Tracheitis
Traumatic reticulitis
Winter dysentery

Table 2.32 Some causes of moderately severe pyrexia: 40.3–41.4°C (104.5–106.5°F)

Anaphylaxis
Anthrax
Aspergillus pneumonia (calves)
Aujeszky's disease
Bacillary haemoglobinuria
Blackleg
Bovine viral diarrhoea
Clostridium perfringens type D
Colisepticaemia (calves)
Contagious bovine pleuropneumonia
Enzootic pneumonia (calves)
Fever
Foot-and-mouth disease
Haemophilus somnus infection
Hypomagnesaemia
Kale poisoning
Laryngitis
Leptospira hardjo infection (septicaemia – early)
Leptospirosis
Liver abscess necrobacillosis (acute)
Lungworm infestation
Meningitis
Mucosal disease
Myositis
Pain
Pericarditis
Peritonitis, acute diffuse
Pneumonia
Pulmonary abscess
Pyrexia/pruritus/haemorrhagic syndrome
Rabies
Salmonella (acute enteritis)
Selenium/vitamin E deficiency (subacute)
Septicaemia
Tetanus
Tickborne fever
Toxaemia
Tracheitis
Traumatic hepatitis
Traumatic pericarditis
Traumatic splenitis

but fluctuating no more than the normal variation, i.e. 1°C (2°F). The temperature remains high for several days before falling with recovery or death.

2. Transient and ephemeral fever. The fever is again present but the rectal temperature only remains high for about a day or less.

Table 2.33 Some causes of severe pyrexia: 41.4–41.9°C (106.5–107.5°F)

Anthrax
Bovine malignant catarrh
Bracken poisoning
Diphtheria (laryngeal)
Fever
Gas gangrene
Haemophilus somnus infection
Heat stroke
Hyperthermia
Infectious bovine rhinotracheitis
Louping ill
Malignant oedema
Metaldehyde poisoning
Peritonitis, acute diffuse
Pharyngeal phlegmon
Photosensitization (severe)
Pneumonia
Redwater fever
Rinderpest
Salmonella septicaemia
Septicaemia

Table 2.34 Pyrexia: some causes of fluctuation

Chronic suppurative pneumonia
Contagious bovine pyelonephritis
Pulmonary ascites
Tuberculosis (*Mycobacterium bovis*)

3. Continuous fever. The temperature remains high for a long period. This raised level is known as the plateau temperature.
4. Intermittent fever. The temperature is high during part of the day but there are non-febrile intervals. The febrile bouts are often regular in occurrence.
5. Remittent fever. The temperature remains high but there are marked fluctuations in the level with differences of more than 1°C (2°F) at short or longer intervals. Often these intervals are irregular.
6. Recurrent fever. This involves long bouts of high temperature, lasting several days, followed by long periods of normal temperature.

7. Undulant fever. This involves long, irregular bouts of high fever, interspersed with similar periods of normal temperature or mild fever.
8. Relapsing fever. The temperature slowly rises to a high level and then immediately falls, only to rise again with the process being repeated on several occasions.
9. Atypical fever. This fever has no regular characteristics and runs an irregular course.

Skin temperature
The surface temperature can be assessed by palpating the animal. This involves feeling the ears, horns, neck, trunk and then passing along to the extremities of the front and hind limbs. Usually the temperature of the ears, limb extremities and base of the tail feel colder than the neck or trunk due to their poorer blood supply. Skin temperature is dependent on the degree of surface capillary dilatation, and is influenced by the heat regulatory centres in the hypothalamus as well as the environmental temperature. However, it can be confusing that the skin may feel cold during the initial stage of fever (the onset). In addition, different areas of the body may show a variation in temperature and this may be due to acute fever, poor circulation, collapse, or muscle rigor. Skin temperature does however rise all over following exertion, muscular activity or exposure to a hot environmental temperature.

Pulse

The pulse is usually palpated in the middle coccygeal artery about 10 cm (4 in) below the anus, the external maxillary (facial) artery on the lateral aspect of the mandible or the median artery on the cranial part of the inside of the forelimb. Various characteristics can be determined, including the frequency, amplitude and rhythm. In obese or excitable animals it might be difficult to feel the pulse and it then can be determined by auscultation of the heart with a stethoscope.

Rate	*Normal resting pulse rate/min*
Cattle	50– 80
Young calves	100–120

The pulse rate is dependent on heart rate and is not significantly affected by local peripheral changes. It tends to vary in normal animals and generally the smaller the animal the higher its pulse rate. The frequency is also higher in younger cattle and following physical exertion. Usually the pulse rate is slightly lower in the male than the female. There is an increased frequency during pregnancy and this becomes even greater as calving approaches. Lactating animals have a higher pulse rate and it is also increased in excitement. The rate tends to be lower in cattle resting in the recumbent position than when standing. The pulse can go up considerably after a meal and is also raised

Table 2.35 Some causes of heart rate over 80/min

Abomasal impaction
Abomasal ulceration
Acidosis
Anaemia
Babesiasis
Bovine viral diarrhoea
Circulation failure, peripheral
Displaced abomasum (left-sided, some cases)
Displaced abomasum (right-sided, some cases)
Downer cow
Encephalitis
Endocarditis
Enzootic bovine leukosis (cardiac form)
Fat cow syndrome (beef, late signs dairy)
Fever
Haemorrhage
Hormone weedkiller poisoning
Mucosal disease
Myocardial weakness
Myopathy
Oleander poisoning (some cases)
Parturient paresis (early stages)
Pericarditis
Peritonitis, acute diffuse
Photosensitization
Pleurisy
Pneumonia
Pulmonary congestion
Pulmonary oedema
Pyrexia
Redwater fever
Septicaemia
Shock
Sporadic bovine leukosis (some cases)
Toxaemia
Traumatic hepatitis
Traumatic reticulitis
Traumatic splenitis
Vagal indigestion (ruminal atony – late stages)

slightly during rumination. High environmental temperatures will result in an increase and this also occurs at low temperatures. Besides these normal alterations in heart rate, increases occur following abnormalities. Thus tachycardia or increased heart rate (Table 2.35, 2.36) follows fever, pain, toxaemia, circulatory failure and excitement. Bradycardia or a decreased rate (Table 2.37) can be seen in partial or complete heart block, space-occupying lesions in the brain, organophosphorus poisoning, or adhesions of the diaphragm in traumatic reticulitis, as well as approaching death.

Table 2.36 Some causes of rapid heart rate (over 100/min)

Abomasal impaction (severe cases)
Abomasal torsion
Acidosis
Anaemia
Anthrax
Arsenic poisoning
Babesiasis
Bacillary haemoglobinuria
Blackleg
Bovine malignant catarrh
Cereal engorgement
Fever (some cases)
Fog fever
Haemorrhage
Heart failure (acute)
Hydrocyanic acid poisoning
Hypomagnesaemia
Intestinal obstruction, acute (if blood vessel occlusion)
Kale poisoning
Leptospirosis (acute)
Lungworm infestation (acute)
Mercury poisoning
Nitrate/nitrite poisoning
Oxalate poisoning (acute)
Parasitic gastroenteritis
Parturient paresis (later stages)
Peritonitis, acute diffuse
Pharyngeal phlegmon
Post-parturient haemoglobinuria
Pyrexia
Redwater fever
Rinderpest
Ruminal tympany
Salmonellosis (acute enteritis)
Selenium/vitamin E deficiency (acute cases)
Septicaemia (some cases)
Traumatic pericarditis
Traumatic reticulitis (if acute diffuse peritonitis)

Table 2.37 Some causes of slow heart rate

Bracken poisoning (calves)
Colienteritis (calves, terminal)
Diaphragmatic hernia
Enteric toxaemia (*Escherichia coli* – calves)
Heart failure (acute)
Hydrocephalus
Nephrosis
Oleander poisoning (some cases)
Organophosphorus poisoning
Traumatic reticulitis
Vagal indigestion (rumen hypermotility)

Rhythm

This is assessed by determining the time interval between each successive pulse wave. These time relationships may be regular or irregular. Rhythm is made up of two components, the amplitude of the pulse waves and the time interval between peaks of the pulse wave. All irregularities should be considered abnormal except sinus arrhythmia where the irregularity coincides with the respiratory cycle. Regular intermittence is rare in cattle but can occur in fit, muscular young cattle and usually disappears with exercise. It is much more common in horses and dogs. Regular irregularities occur with a constant time interval and are usually associated with partial heart block. Irregular irregularities obviously occur without any pattern and are usually associated with variations in the stroke volume of the blood. The usual causes are either ventricular extrasystolic arrhythmias or atrial fibrillations. Pulse irregularities tend to disappear with exercise except in the case of auricular fibrillation when they become accentuated. The significance of such pulse irregularities is that they indicate myocardial disease.

Amplitude

The amplitude or pulse quality is difficult to determine and depends on assessing the amount of digital pressure to obliterate the pulse wave in the artery. The amplitude varies because the rate of diastolic filling of the heart influences the stroke volume. Changes in the pulse character can be the result of structural or functional disease of the heart, or they may be the indirect effect of blood vessel abnormalities such as venous congestion or vasomotor disturbance. The amplitude can be considerably increased in aortic semilunar valve incompetence

Table 2.38 Some causes of reduced/weak pulse

Anaemia
Arsenic poisoning
Bacillary haemoglobinuria
Circulation failure, peripheral
Dehydration
Fever
Foot-and-mouth disease (cardiac form)
Heat stroke
Heart failure, acute (absent)
Hydrocyanic acid poisoning (subacute)
Hyperthermia
Nephrosis
Nitrate/nitrite poisoning
Parturient paresis
Pyrexia
Salmonellosis (acute enteritis)
Septicaemia
Shock (weak)
Toxaemia
Traumatic pericarditis

where there is a 'water hammer' pulse. There is a decrease in amplitude in most cases of myocardial weakness (Table 2.38).

Examination of the mucous membranes

Observation of the mucous membranes usually indicates the quality and condition of the circulatory system. The normal mucous membranes which can be checked easily are the conjunctivae, the mouth, nostrils, vulva and possibly rectum. Observations must be performed in good lighting, preferably daylight. There can be various alterations, especially in colour, discharges, swellings or haemorrhages.

Colour

Where an abnormal colour is seen in one area, other areas should be checked to see if they also show the change. If only one area is affected then the problem is localized or is just a peculiarity of the particular animal. Likewise if one conjunctiva or nostril mucosa is abnormal then the other should also be inspected. Pale mucous membranes are indicative of shock or anaemia (Table 2.39). When severe the lack of colour results in membranes turning grey-white to white. This paleness may be acute as occurs following shock, and haemorrhage, or chronic as with paratuberculosis (Johne's disease) or tuberculosis.

Table 2.39 Some causes of pale mucous membranes

Anaemia
Circulation failure, peripheral
Cobalt deficiency
Copper deficiency
Copper poisoning (chronic)
Displaced abomasum (right-sided)
Endocarditis
Enteric toxaemia (*Escherichia coli* calves)
Enzootic haematuria
Fascioliasis
Haemonchosis
Haemorrhage
Heart failure, acute
Johne's disease
Kale poisoning
Leptospirosis (acute)
Nitrate/nitrite poisoning
Parasitic gastroenteritis (Ostertagia type II)
Post-parturient haemoglobinuria
Ragwort poisoning
Redwater fever (mid stages)
Shock
Thrombosis of vena cava
Tuberculosis

Redness is the result of congestion with distended blood vessels (Table 2.40). When severe the colour may become brick-red. This can be seen in shipping fever, malignant catarrhal fever and infectious bovine keratoconjunctivitis. A reddish colour due to venous congestion occurs in pulmonary disease, pneumonia, pleurisy, heart disease, endocarditis, traumatic pericarditis. A dark brick-red colour resembling haemorrhage occurs in severe, usually fatal, disease. Cyanosis (Table 2.41) is not common but results in a dark reddish-blue colour and is seen in respiratory insufficiency.

In many cattle it is very difficult to determine if an animal shows icterus in its early stages. This can also be complicated by the breed involved.

Jaundice (Table 2.42) can occur and results initially in dirty-coloured membranes but if the animal is anaemic then the colour is usually a yellowish-white or golden. This can occur in cases of haemolytic anaemia as with babesiasis, and liver problems such as ragwort poisoning. Yellow discoloration can occur naturally in the mucous membranes of Channel Island and South Devon cattle.

Table 2.40 Some causes of red mucous membranes

Anthrax (congested)
Arsenic poisoning
Hydrocyanic acid poisoning (bright red)
Infectious bovine rhinotracheitis
Pulmonary congestion (bright red – nasal)
Pulmonary oedema (bright red – nasal)
Redwater fever (early stages)
Rhinitis (nasal)
Rinderpest
Salmonella (acute enteritis)
Summer snuffles (nasal)

Table 2.41 Some causes of cyanosis

Anaphylaxis (severe)
Congestive heart failure (left)
Hydrocyanic acid poisoning
Metaldehyde poisoning
Nitrate/nitrite poisoning
Patent foramen ovale (calf)
Pneumonia (unusual sign)
Tetralogy of Fallot (calf)

Table 2.42 Some causes of jaundice

Bacillary haemoglobinuria
Carbon tetrachloride poisoning
Copper poisoning (chronic)
Endocarditis
Hepatitis
Kale poisoning
Leptospirosis
Lupinosis
Phenothiazine poisoning
Phosphorus poisoning
Photosensitization
Post-parturient haemoglobinuria
Ragwort poisoning

Spotted or faint reddening of the mucous membranes is nearly always due to haemorrhages. Petechial and ecchymotic haemorrhages (Table 2.43) can occur in leptospirosis, anthrax, bracken poisoning and shipping fever as well as colibacillosis in calves.

Table 2.43 Some causes of mucous membrane haemorrhages

Anthrax (acute)
Bracken poisoning
Copper poisoning (acute)
Leptospirosis (acute)
Mycotoxicosis
Pyrexia/pruritus/haemorrhagic syndrome
Sweet vernal grass poisoning

Discharge

This can be from one or all mucosal orifices. Where only one set of membranes is involved it is likely that the condition is localized. In addition, it can be either unilateral or bilateral. The former again indicates a localized problem. The discharge can be serous, mucous, mucopurulent or purulent. The amount of discharge also varies. Discharge from the eyes (Table 2.44) does not occur in healthy cattle although excessive lachrymation (epiphora) can occur following irritation in the environment such as dust, bright sun, insects and wind. Serous discharges from the eyes and nose are common in infectious bovine rhinotracheitis, mucosal disease and rinderpest. When only one conjunctiva is affected it is more likely to be infectious bovine keratoconjunctivitis. Purulent discharge may be seen in rinderpest, infectious bovine rhinotracheitis, mucosal disease and

Table 2.44 Some causes of ocular discharge

Blue tongue
Bovine viral diarrhoea
Bovine malignant catarrh
Bracken poisoning (some)
Cobalt deficiency (late stages)
Conjunctival foreign body
Contagious bovine pleuropneumonia
Cuffing pneumonia (calves, mucopurulent)
Dusty feed rhinotracheitis
Enzootic pneumonia (calves, mucopurulent)
Infectious bovine keratoconjunctivitis
Infectious bovine rhinotracheitis
Mucosal disease
Parasitic bronchitis (some)
Pasteurellosis (pneumonic – mucopurulent)
Rinderpest
Summer snuffles (mucopurulent)
Vitamin A deficiency (mucoid)

malignant catarrhal fever. Chronic discharge, particularly epiphora, results in loss of hair under the medial canthus of the eye. Nasal discharges are listed in Table 6.1.

Swelling

Swelling of the mucous membranes is seen uncommonly. It does however often occur in the conjunctiva or vulva. If severe, the mucosa can protrude out from the eye. Vulval swellings often occur around or following parturition. In the acute form swellings can be seen in anthrax, rinderpest and malignant catarrhal fever. Chronic swelling exists in chronic fascioliasis, parasitic bronchitis and haemonchosis.

Haemorrhages

Generalized mucosal haemorrhages are very rare in cattle but can occur in leptospirosis, the later stages of anthrax and bracken poisoning. Localized haemorrhages can be the result of trauma or other damage, or occasionally following severe infections.

Odours

An acute sense of smell is of assistance to the veterinary surgeon. Various odours can be of considerable use in making a diagnosis. They may involve the animal itself or its environment. The characteristic acrid smell of calf scour is always useful, especially when scour is not obviously present. Acetonaemia results in an acetone or pear-drop smell on the breath and the animal. A sweet–sour smell may occur with acidosis. Purulent odours can occur in cases of bronchial disease, infectious pododermatitis, endometritis, etc. A fetid or putrid smell may be present if necrosis occurs and it can be found around the head in severe infectious bovine rhinotracheitis or oral necrobacillosis. It is also apparent in gangrenous cases of mastitis.

Examination of the lymph nodes

Lymph nodes may become enlarged (Table 2.45), when they are often visible and palpable. This enlargement is seen in disease and neoplasia. When swollen they may be painful in acute problems and hard in chronic inflammation. Only a few of the major lymph nodes can be palpated in normal cattle; other nodes can be palpated when enlarged. In other areas swelling of

Table 2.45 Some causes of enlarged lymph nodes

Actinobacillosis
Atypical *Mycobacterium* infection
Bovine malignant catarrh
Enzootic bovine leukosis
Infections (generalized or localized)
Neoplasia (generalized or localized)
Septicaemia
Sporadic bovine leukosis
Tuberculosis (avian)
Tuberculosis (bovine)

the lymph nodes results in obstruction and can lead to bloat, dyspnoea or asphyxiation. Those which can normally be felt (Figure 2.1) are:

Submandibular or submaxillary

This is found between the sternocephalicus muscle and the ventral parts of the mandibular salivary gland. The gland is oval and in some cases there is a second gland which may vary in position.

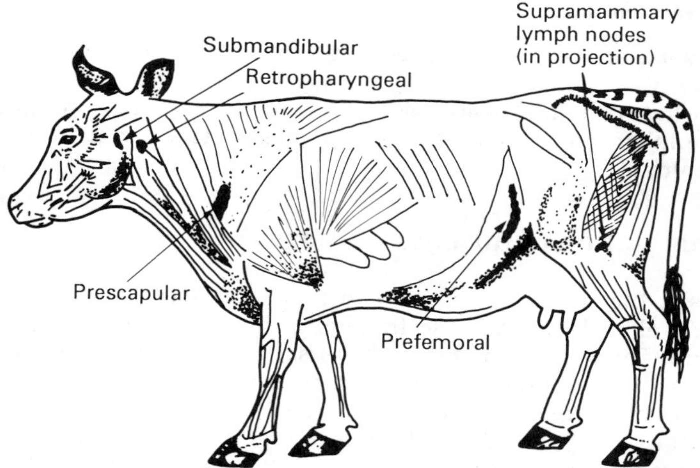

Figure 2.1 Superficial lymphatic glands. (Supermammary glands in projection). From *Diagnostic Methods in Veterinary Medicine*, 6th edition, G.F. Boddie. Edinburgh, Oliver & Boyd

Suprapharyngeal (retropharyngeal)

These are difficult to palpate in the healthy animal. They can be found above the larynx and are felt by pushing hard with the fingers in the caudal pharyngeal region.

Prescapular

This is in the subcutaneous tissue about 10–12 cm (4–5 in) above the shoulder. It is elongated and can often most easily be felt by pushing the fingers caudally towards the cranial border of the scapula.

Prefemoral (precrural)

This is the largest superficial node in the cow. It is on the cranial border of the tensor fasciae latae about 10 cm (4 in) above the patella and is readily palpable and moveable.

Superficial inguinal

In the bull they are in the mass of fat above the scrotal neck and caudal to the spermatic cord.

Supramammary

They are above the caudal border of the udder and are two in number.

Rectal palpation can allow the rectal, internal inguinal, sublumbar, internal iliac and mesenteric lymph nodes to be examined.

Examination of the environment

This is the third part of the clinical examination and again is essential in both the case involving the single animal or the group. The reasons are more obvious in the latter instance, but it is equally true in the former as it may provide essential evidence on the cause of the problem, as well as influencing advice on control and prevention. Often the animal will have been removed from others within the group and so a point should be made of looking at where it came from. This also allows examination of the rest of the group to see if the problem has spread. Most benefit can be obtained from such an investigation

Table 2.46 Some factors to be considered when examining the environment

Indoors
Group size
Space allowances
Ventilation
Bedding
Disinfection procedures
Drainage
Flooring
Cattle movements
Light
Other buildings
Method of feeding/water provision
Reproduction management
Outdoors
Position
Soil type
Stocking level
Grassland management
Fertilizer usage
Plant types
Climate
Shelter
Feed supplements
Water supply

by those who have a satisfactory knowledge of animal husbandry and production.

Environment can be divided most easily into the indoor environment and that outside. Generally more problems occur in housed conditions and so these will be dealt with first.

Indoors

Cattle were designed by nature as grazing animals to make use of grass and other forms of herbage for their maintenance and growth. They are adapted to an outside environment and are able to cope well provided they are given the freedom to seek shelter when necessary and are in an area supplied with adequate nutrition and water.

When cattle come indoors they are in an abnormal environment. They tend to be grouped together in large numbers, often with limited floor and air space per animal. This means that there is a good opportunity for infectious agents to spread between the cattle, it also allows increased problems with the pecking order and at times it can lead to abnormal behaviour.

Cattle which have been used to the rigours of an inclement outside environment or those being fed for maximum growth have particular problems in adapting to an enclosed environment. When examining the environment it is essential to look for overcrowding, poor accommodation and bad ventilation for the group from which the animal came as well as for the building in general.

Space allowances

Space allowances for cattle are known and can be judged by eye within the group. What is equally important is the number in the group and their access to feed and water.

Ventilation

Ventilation needs to be assessed, both in terms of the building and the number of animals within the particular air space. When ventilation is inadequate it predisposes to respiratory conditions but also stresses the animals so that they become more susceptible to other conditions. Too humid an environment will help to keep the coats of the animals wet and then other problems can result. Humid conditions are usually indicated by wet ceilings, walls or bedding. The presence of many cobwebs also indicates little air movement. If fans are used, their position and how they are regulated may be important as well as trying to detect the presence of draughts. Too dry or dusty an environment can also predispose to an increase in respiratory problems.

Bedding

Drainage and bedding need to be assessed to see that the animals are kept clean and dry without excessive humidity. The bedding or flooring should be sufficient to maintain the animals in a dry state and keep their access to faeces and potential pathogens to a minimum.

Disinfection procedures

It is important to know how often cleaning is undertaken and what it involves, i.e. depopulation, washing and disinfection, and when it was last done in relation to the present problem. The proper physical removal of faeces, and leaving the house depopulated, are far better disinfectants than relying on chemicals in partly-cleared buildings. The type of bedding may be important in disease, particularly in problems such as mastitis and lameness.

Drainage

Poor drainage can lead to a build-up of ammonia and other gases, again predisposing to trouble, as well as often indicating both drainage and ventilation problems.

Overcrowding and poor faecal disposal can lead to considerable problems with dirty cattle and skin conditions. This in turn may result in other problems.

Flooring

Flooring is particularly important and the presence of slippery surfaces or poorly laid or maintained concrete can lead to trouble. Although slatted floors may work well, they can also lead to locomotory conditions and soiling of the animals.

Cattle movements

In contagious disease it is often important to look at the movements of cattle and other animals to ensure minimum spread. Contact between individuals and groups also needs to be assessed.

Light

The degree of light available in the building is important not only on welfare grounds but also in the ability of the stockman to undertake his routine procedures and observe animals.

Other buildings

Mastitis problems obviously involve examination of the milking parlour, milking routine and milking machine. However, it is important not to overlook how the animals are housed and managed.

Method of feeding/water provision

Feeding is usually mechanical and can involve providing each individual feed or mixing them. The latter leaves more room for error, particularly if more than one person is involved or someone different takes over at weekends or holidays. Self-feed silage can produce difficulties if there is not sufficient silage face or if provision has not been made for heifers entering the herd. Over-impacted silage may be difficult to remove particularly for heifers erupting permanent front teeth or older cows. Examination of the silage face may show selective feeding, usually due to areas of poor quality which may contain high butyric acid levels or be mouldy.

Reproduction management

Where bulls are involved their accommodation and situation in relation to the rest of the herd should be noted. Where there are abortions or reproductive problems it is necessary to know whether natural or artificial insemination is used. The provisions made for service need to be assessed as also does the area for insemination. The provision of calving boxes and how they are cleaned between occupants may be important in mastitis, metritis problems as well as in calf scour. Knowledge of the breeding policy may be necessary if conditions are thought to be congenital. Management of reproduction, identification and records will need to be included when dealing with breeding problems.

Outdoors

Position

The positioning of the farm, whether in an exposed situation or in a valley, can alter the disease problems encountered. There may or may not be adequate shelter and if woodland is present it may predispose to summer mastitis and infectious bovine keratoconjunctivitis. The presence of natural water sources on the farm may result in contamination and problems such as salmonellosis, fascioliasis, anthrax or possible toxin problems. Brackish water or ponds used for drinking can help disseminate conditions such as Johne's disease, salmonellosis and fascioliasis. The position of the fields in relation to the farm buildings is important. There is always a tendency for animals not to be observed properly the further they are from the main buildings. Thus if disease occurs it may often be at an advanced stage before it is noticed.

Neighbouring areas can make a difference, such as the presence of a sewage works or factories. These can possibly lead to infections or toxic conditions. Proximity to lay-bys or housing developments can lead to problems such as poisoning, particularly with lead but also plants, as well as *Cysticercus bovis*. The boundary fences are also important in determining the possibility of animals escaping or entering the farm and thereby disseminating disease. They are also indicative of whether disease is likely to spread from farm to farm, as with warble fly, tuberculosis and lungworm infection.

Soil type

The type of soil is important in that it may be responsible for deficiencies such as those of selenium, copper or cobalt. However, toxicity problems such as molybdenosis, arsenic and lead poisoning can also occur. Hopefully when investigating the history, indications will have been given as to whether additional feeding has alleviated or exacerbated the problem. The soil type can also influence problems, such as a heavy clay resulting in adherence of soil to the feet. Dry, hard land can lead to bruising of the sole and interdigital pododermatitis. Poor quality soil and herbage form suitable habitats for ectoparasites such as the tick, *Ixodes ricinus*.

Stocking level

As with conditions indoors, cattle can be overcrowded at pasture. The level of stocking must depend on the amount of forage available plus any supplementary feeding being provided and the required rate of production. Where conditions are overcrowded they predispose to deficiency problems and also poisonings, particularly by plants. Higher stocking levels are acceptable where there is adequate grassland management. Where this is not practised there will be a concentration of faeces and thereby potential infections such as parasitic gastroenteritis, parasitic bronchitis, Johne's disease, etc.

Grassland management

Good grassland management is a method of improving the feed value of pasture as well as improving stocking rate and decreasing potential disease problems. Even where set stocking is used, the proper use of fertilizer will increase grass growth and thereby dilute potential problems with parasitic gastroenteritis and parasitic bronchitis. The use of rotational grazing, mixed stocking, leader–follower, ⅓–⅔, and 1, 2, 3 systems together with planned anthelmintic usage all help improve growth and reduce helminth problems. Provision of a lush pasture in the autumn to suckler cows can predispose to fog fever. Grazing poor quality dead grass in the autumn can lead to problems such as vitamin A deficiency and hypomagnesaemia.

Fertilizer usage

Good fertilizer usage helps reduce problems. Thus delaying the use of potash in the spring will reduce hypomagnesaemia; liming will often increase deficiencies of copper and cobalt. However, increasing the alkalinity of the soil increases selenium uptake by plants and also reduces the incidence of clinical Johne's disease.

Plant types

The composition of the sward has effects on certain problems. Clover tends to reduce hypomagnesaemia but increase ruminal tympany. The old breeds of grass, often nowadays thought to be of poor quality, tend to have high levels of minerals and to reduce metabolic problems such as hypomagnesaemia. The use of sainfoin allows access to high protein levels without bloat.

Climate

Changes in climate can produce problems. A change to damp, muggy conditions in the autumn or spring can result in pasteurellosis outside or enzootic pneumonia in calves indoors. Warm, humid weather in the spring predisposes to frothy bloat. Sudden severe frosts or wet weather in spring or autumn can precipitate grass tetany outbreaks.

Shelter

Cattle should always have access to some form of shelter, even if only a windbreak. It is when this is lacking that losses from hypomagnesaemia can be high in adults and outbreaks of diarrhoea in calves will be severe with high morbidity and mortality.

Feed supplements

When supplementation of the pasture is undertaken it is important to know how much is fed and to be sure in one's own mind that all the animals have equal access to it. If prevention of staggers or bloat involves feeding roughage prior to grazing it is important to know that the feed has in fact been eaten prior to going out to grass. Buffer silage feeding at pasture to reduce milk fever must also be available to all dry cows. Feed can occasionally be the source of infectious or toxic agents.

Water supply

The origin of the water supply, whether natural or mains, needs to be known. It is also important to ascertain that sufficient is always available. This is particularly so in the summer months with dairy cattle. Where supplies are unreliable, the storage provisions for water should be known. Water may be necessary as a vehicle for treatment, or more likely prevention of disease. Water, like feed, can occasionally be contaminated with potential pathogens or toxins.

3 Alimentary system

Prehension
Mastication
Pica
Stomatitis
Pharyngitis
Pharyngeal obstruction
Salivation
Deglutition (swallowing)
Oesophagus
Regurgitation
Reticulorumen
Ruminal atony
Ruminal tympany
Abomasal dilatation
Abomasitis
Intestinal obstruction
Alimentary dilatation
Enteritis
Peritonitis
Constipation
Tenesmus
Diarrhoea (differential diagnosis)
Colic

Prehension

Usually feed is drawn into the mouth by the tongue and then nipped off between the front teeth and the dental pad (Table 3.1). Drinking involves sucking up water with the tongue producing a negative vacuum in the mouth. This can be interfered with but is not a common problem. It can follow paralysis of the muscles of the lips, tongue or jaws. Usually with nervous disease paralysis is seen with affected muscles showing flaccidity (listeriosis) or marked rigidity (tetanus). Often these animals will appear to want to eat but they are unable to do so. Problems are few without other organs being affected and many cases are due to painful foci in the mouth (Table 3.2). When the tongue is painful cattle may try to prehend with their lips.

Table 3.1 Causes of absent or reduced prehension

General infections	Tetanus, listeriosis, rabies
Anatomical problems	Malformation of the jaw, teeth; malapposition of the upper and lower mandibles
Trauma	Mandible or mucosae
Local infection	Osteomyelitis of mandible, infection of mucosae, stomatitis, glossitis
Buccal pain	Foreign body in the mouth, fluorosis

Table 3.2 Some causes of mouth lesions

Actinobacillosis
Actinomycosis
Aujeszky's disease (calf)
Blue tongue
Bovine malignant catarrh
Bovine papular stomatitis
Bovine viral diarrhoea
Diphtheria (necrobacillosis, calf)
Foot-and-mouth disease
Mercury poisoning (petechiation and tender gingiva)
Mucosal disease
Rinderpest
Stomatitis
Zinc deficiency (ulcer on dental pad, haemorrhages around teeth)

Mastication

Problems with mastication are few but can arise and usually they are local in origin (Table 3.3). Thus examination of the region will usually reveal the cause of the problem. In some animals cuds will be dropped while eating. In other cases cuds are retained in the mouth, usually in an area of ulceration or inflammation (e.g. calf diphtheria). The faeces also tend to contain large quantities of undigested food, largely fibrous in nature. When the mouth is very painful the animal will make no attempt to chew.

Table 3.3 Causes of absent or reduced mastication

Tooth abnormalities	Front or cheek tooth eruption (calves or growing cattle) Loss of teeth (older cattle) Peridontal disease
Infections	Stomatitis, glossitis, osteomyelitis Calf diphtheria Foot-and-mouth disease, malignant catarrhal fever, mucosal disease
Trauma	Jaws, buccal or glossal mucosae

Pica (allotriophagia, depraved appetite)

Cases of depraved appetite are relatively rare in cattle but do occur (Table 3.4) and are usually the result of a nutritional problem, e.g. lack of roughage in the diet. This condition may be associated with excessive licking and some cases of pica are the result of boredom but this is unusual.

Stomatitis (Table 3.5)

This is a general term covering inflammation of the oral mucosa. Included in the definition is inflammation of the mucosa of the tongue (glossitis), hard palate (palatitis) and gums (gingivitis).

Pharyngitis (Table 3.6)

Localized inflammation of the pharynx is rare in cattle, although it often forms part of more generalized infections.

Table 3.4 Causes of pica, excessive licking and urine drinking

Pica
Infections
- Abomasitis
- Actinomycosis
- Rabies

Nutritional
- Acetonaemia
- Cobalt deficiency (unusual)
- Copper deficiency (unusual)
- Lack of roughage
- Phosphorus deficiency
- Post-parturient haemoglobinuria
- Selenium poisoning (chronic)
- Sodium chloride deficiency
- Vitamin D deficiency (young cattle)

Excessive licking
Deficiencies
- Acetonaemia (nervous)
- Boredom
- Lack of roughage
- Salt deficiency
- Water deprivation

Urine drinking
- Boredom (usually calves)
- Salt deficiency
- Water deprivation

Table 3.5 Some causes of stomatitis

Physical	Foreign bodies, trauma, balling or drenching damage, inexpert gagging, abrasive fibre, sharp grass or cereal awns, malocclusion of teeth, differential tooth wear, tooth loss, eating hot food, drinking hot water, eating frozen food
Chemicals	Irritant chemicals such as acids, alkalis, chloral hydrate, mercury
Infections	*Bacterial*: calf diphtheria, actinomycosis, actinobacillosis *Viral*: bovine papular stomatitis, blue tongue, rinderpest, vesicular stomatitis, foot-and-mouth disease, malignant catarrhal fever, mucosal disease, upper alimentary squamous cell carcinoma *Fungal*: *Monilia* spp., *Nocardia* spp.

Pharyngeal obstruction

This is very uncommon in cattle but can occasionally follow neglected chronic infections or physical problems (Table 3.7).

Table 3.6 Some causes of pharyngitis

Physical	Grass or cereal awns, foreign bodies, inexpert tubing, eating hot food, drinking hot water, eating frozen food
Chemical	Irritant chemicals such as acids, alkalis, chloral hydrate, mercury
Infections	*Bacterial*: Actinobacillosis, *Fusiformis necrophorus*, 'pharyngeal phlegmon' (possibly *Fusiformis necrophorus*)
	Often associated with stomatitis or upper respiratory tract infections

Table 3.7 Some causes of pharyngeal obstruction

Physical	Large foreign bodies, e.g. potatoes, placental membranes
Infections	Enlarged retropharyngeal lymph nodes, actinobacillosis, tuberculosis, enzootic bovine leukosis, sporadic bovine leukosis
Lesions	Enlarged retropharyngeal lymph nodes, polyps (fibrous, mucoid), diffuse pharyngeal enlargement, soft palate enlargement

Salivation

Increased salivation can be the result of increased saliva production or the absence or reduction in the rate of swallowing, or a response to pain or inflammation (Table 3.8). A decrease occurs in fever, dehydration or other problems which reduce secretory flow, e.g. parturition paresis.

Deglutition (swallowing)

The act of conveying food and water from the mouth, through the pharynx to the oesophagus and thence the reticulorumen is very complex. The posterior part of the tongue pushes the food towards the oesophagus. Closure of the exits in the pharynx creates pressure to allow the food or fluid into the oesophagus. Food passes along the oesophagus by peristalsis whereas liquid slides down the oesophagus. This complicated procedure involves reflex actions controlled by several nerves including the trigeminal (V), glossopharyngeal (IX), laryngeal (X) and hypoglossal (XII).

Table 3.8 Some causes of increased salivation

Actinomycosis
Arsenic poisoning
Aujeszky's disease
Blue tongue
Botulism
Bovine malignant catarrh
Bovine viral diarrhoea
Brain abscess (rete mirabile)
Candida spp. poisoning
Cerebrocortical necrosis (frothy)
Chlorinated hydrocarbon poisoning
Clostridium perfringens type D
Coenurosis
Diphtheria (laryngeal)
Diphtheria, calf (stomatitis)
Encephalitis
Foot-and-mouth disease
Frothing at the mouth
Gid
Hormone weedkiller poisoning
Hypomagnesaemia
Infectious bovine rhinotracheitis
Lead poisoning (acute, subacute)
Levamisole poisoning
Listeria infection (meningoencephalitis)
Lupin poisoning (frothy)
Mercury poisoning
Metaldehyde poisoning
Mucosal disease
Nitrate/nitrite poisoning
Oesophageal obstruction
Oesophageal paralysis
Oesophagitis
Organophosphorus poisoning
Penitrem A poisoning
Pharyngeal paralysis
Pharyngeal phlegmon
Pharyngitis
Phosphorus poisoning
Rabies
Riboflavin deficiency
Rickets
Rinderpest (blood-stained, then purulent)
Ruminal tympany
Stomatitis
Tetanus
Water hemlock poisoning (frothy)

Fortunately few problems actually arise from this process but very occasionally pharyngeal paralysis can occur (Table 3.9).

Table 3.9 Some causes of pharyngeal paralysis

Physical	Pressure on local nerve supply – local trauma, suppurative pharyngitis, enlarged lymph nodes, abscessation (actinobacillosis, tuberculosis, enzootic bovine leukosis, sporadic bovine leukosis)
Infections	Encephalitis, botulism, listeriosis, rabies

Oesophagus

The connection between the mouth and reticulorumen again develops few specific problems (Table 3.10). Oesophagitis can occur, as also can oesophageal obstruction.

Table 3.10 Causes of oesophageal problems

Physical	Potatoes, turnips, carrots, mangolds, swedes Laceration of mucosa by sharp foreign bodies Faulty use of stomach tube
Infections	*Viral*: bovine malignant catarrh, mucosal disease, rinderpest *Parasites*: *Hypoderma lineata* larvae
Lesions	Oesophageal stenosis after previous obstruction External pressure from enlarged lymph nodes (tuberculosis, actinobacillosis, enzootic bovine leukosis, sporadic bovine leukosis)

Regurgitation

Food regurgitation is unusual and causes are shown in Table 3.11.

Table 3.11 Regurgitation: food or fluid

Diaphragmatic hernia
Megaoesophagus
Mucosal disease
Oesophagitis
Persistence of the right aortic arch (calf)
Pharyngeal obstruction (mainly via mouth)
Pharyngeal paralysis
Pharyngeal phlegmon (severe cases)
Pharyngitis (severe cases)

Reticulorumen

Ruminants have been adapted to the consumption and digestion of large quantities of grass. This is accomplished by means of bacterial and protozoal digestion of the food in a large fermentation chamber, the reticulorumen. Food from the oesophagus enters the primary compartment of the reticulorumen. There are three forestomachs, the rumen (first), reticulum (second) and omasum (third) before reaching the fourth or true stomach (abomasum) (Figures 3.1 and 3.2). In the adult the rumen is by far the longest and has a capacity of about 80% of the four stomach capacities, varying from 135 to 225 litres (30 to

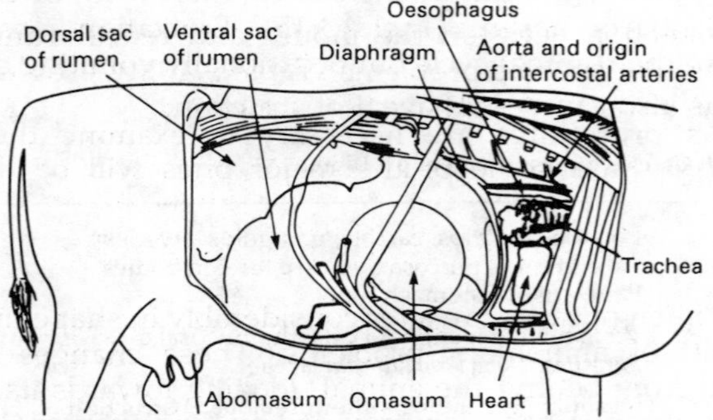

Figure 3.1 Right side of bovine abdomen showing forestomach. From *Clinical Examination of Cattle*, 2nd edition, G. Rosenberger *et al.* (1977). Translated 1979 by R. Mack. Berlin, Verlag

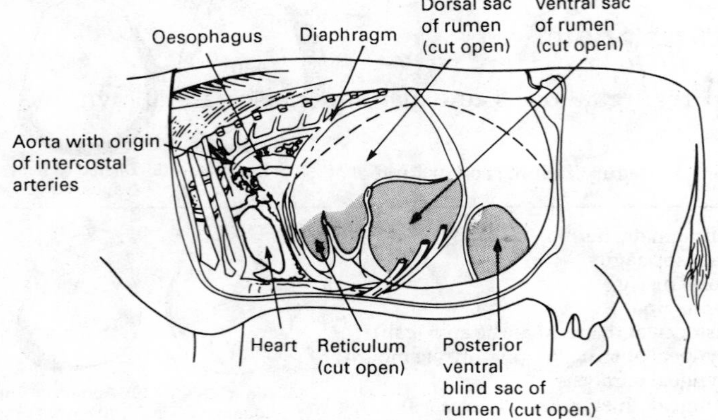

Figure 3.2 Left side of bovine abdomen, rumen cut away. From *Clinical Examination of Cattle*, 2nd edition, G. Rosenberger *et al.* (1977). Translated 1979 by R. Mack. Berlin, Verlag

50 gallons). The reticulum is the smallest of the four stomachs and has a capacity of about 5% of the total with that of the omasum being 8% and the abomasum 7%. In the newborn calf the abomasum is about twice as large as the reticulum and rumen combined but by 10–12 weeks this ratio will have been reversed.

It is important to understand the normal ruminal cycles as these often become disturbed in digestive problems (Table 3.12). The ruminal cycles are concerned with mixing feed, eructating gas and expelling cuds to the mouth. The waves of movement occur at regular intervals which alter with the type of feed present in the rumen. There are usually about two cycles per minute. Movements can be increased (Table 3.13) or decreased (Table 3.14), or absent (Table 3.15). Eructation is a normal process in the ruminal cycle but occasionally vomiting can occur (Table 3.16).

Various procedures are necessary to examine the rumen satisfactorily and some of the major ones will be discussed briefly.

Inspection

The abdomen of cattle can alter considerably in shape, mainly as the result of alimentary problems. These changes are best observed from behind the animal, looking towards its head. A useful description has been provided by Rosenberger (1977) and it forms the basis of this discussion (Figure 3.3). Occasionally there is a reduction in ruminal size (Table 3.17).

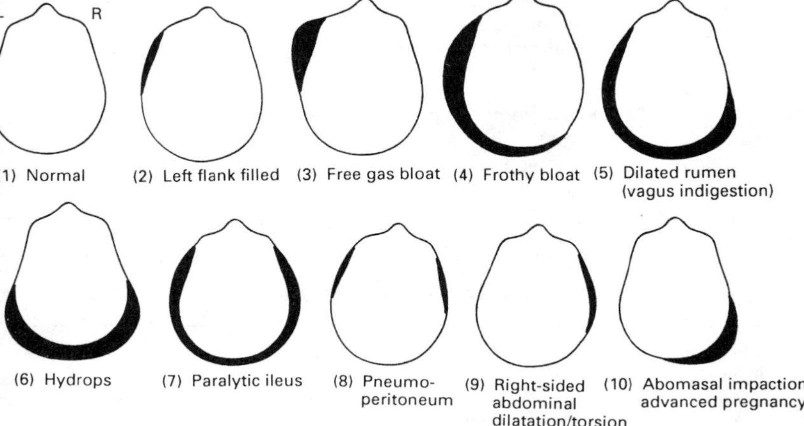

Figure 3.3 Diagram of the abdominal outline (seen from behind) of some problems. From G. Rosenberger *et al.* (1977), *Medical examination of cattle*, 2nd edition (translated 1979 by R. Mack), Berlin, Verlag.

Table 3.12 Stages of the rumination cycle

Ruminal cycle	*Reticulorumen*	*Omasum*
Stage 1	Two contractions of reticulum and reticuloruminal fold	Dilatation of omasal canal
Result	Reticular contents pass over reticuloruminal fold into rumen	Passage of feed into the omasum
Stage 2	Contraction of ruminal atrium, dorsal blind sac and ruminal pillar	Contraction of omasal canal
Result	Movement of reticular fluid over reticuloruminal fold into relaxed rumen	Transport of feed from omasal canal into omasum
	Passage of coarse particles over the ruminal pillar into dorsal blind sac	
	Movement of dorsal sac results in squeezing and mixing of solid contents	
Stage 3	Contraction of ventral sac and pillar of rumen with relaxation of dorsal sac	Contraction of omasum
Result	Fluid part of rumen contents returns to dorsal sac and ruminal atrium and is forced through the fibrous matter	Contents squeezed. Slow removal of contents to abomasum
Stage 4	Contraction of dorsal sac and pillar of rumen	Contraction of omasal canal
Result	Transfer of accumulated gut contents to the cardia resulting in eructation	Emptying of omasal canal
Eructation		
	Reticular contraction prior to stage 1	
	Reticular bolus projected into mouth	

Table 3.13 Some causes of increased ruminal movements

Oesophageal obstruction
Ruminal tympany (early stages)
Tetanus
Vagal indigestion (rumen hypermotility)

Table 3.14 Some causes of depressed ruminal movements

Acetonaemia
Bovine viral diarrhoea (acute)
Cereal engorgement (mild)
Displaced abomasum (left – always amplitude, sometimes frequency)
Indigestion, simple (amplitude and frequency)
Mucosal disease
Oxalate poisoning (acute)
Peritonitis, localized
Pyrexia
Ruminal atony (amplitude and frequency)
Toxaemia
Traumatic reticulitis
Vagal indigestion (some ruminal atony)

Table 3.15 Some causes of absent ruminal movements

Abomasal impaction
Acidosis
Anthrax
Arsenic poisoning
Bacillary haemoglobinuria
Blackleg
Cereal engorgement (severe)
Contagious bovine pleuropneumonia
Diaphragmatic hernia
Displaced abomasum (right-sided – most cases)
Fodder beet poisoning
Gas gangrene
Hormone weedkiller poisoning
Indigestion, simple
Kale poisoning
Lead poisoning
Malignant oedema
Mangel poisoning
Parturient paresis
Peritonitis, localized
Pyrexia
Redwater fever
Ruminal atony
Sugar beet poisoning
Transit tetany
Traumatic reticulitis
Vagal indigestion (pyloric obstruction)
Vagal indigestion (ruminal atony)

Table 3.16 Some causes of vomiting

An unusual sign in cattle but it can follow various problems:
Abomasitis, acute (sometimes)
Arsenic poisoning
Crude oil poisoning
Diaphragmatic hernia (occasionally when examined)
Hydrocyanic acid poisoning (occasionally)
Nitrate/nitrite poisoning
Oesophageal diverticulum
Oesophagitis (mainly regurgitation)
Oleander poisoning
Rhododendron poisoning
Ruminal tympany
Sodium chlorate poisoning

1. Normal outline with roughly symmetrical shape.
2. Left flank slightly distended dorsally with a gaseous consistency. This can occur in (a) stenosis of the oesophageal sphincter, (b) piercing foreign body, (c) extreme left-side displacement of the abomasum, (d) localized peritoneal abscess (after use of trochar and cannula or laparotomy).
3. Semi-bloat (gaseous), usually due to excessive cereal feeding or oesophageal obstruction.
4. Enlargement of most of the left side of the abdomen – usually frothy bloat due to legumes.
5. Moderately relapsing tympany and dilatation of the rumen with functional gaseous stenosis (occurs in vagal indigestion).
6. Ventral abdominal swelling (occurs in ascites, or hydrops amnii, also old cows and bulls).
7. All-round enlargement with a barrel-shaped abdomen (occurs in prolonged ruminal tympany, secondary ruminal tympany, paralytic ileus).
8. Both flanks filled with gas (unusual but can occur with generalized peritonitis with gas formation, abdominal penetration, previous surgery such as laparotomy, trocharization).
9. Right flank filled and slightly bulging (occurs in right-sided abomasal dilatation, torsion of the uterus, torsion of the caecum, intestinal volvulus or early paralytic ileus).

Table 3.17 Some cases of reduction in abdominal size

Chronic	Starvation, malnutrition, deficiency diseases Chronic infections (tuberculosis, liver abscess, chronic peritonitis, pyelonephritis, chronic pneumonia)
Subacute	Severe diarrhoea

10. The ventral part of the right abdominal wall bulging (occurs in simple abomasal dilatation, advanced pregnancy).

Abdominal size reduction

This is less common but can occur in chronic infections such as tuberculosis, chronic pneumonia, or serious subacute disease.

External palpation

This gives an indication of the consistency of the abdominal contents. A tense left-sided abdomen can be due to gas or excessive ruminal filling. Palpation of the rumen may show the contents to be 'doughy' or to appear very fluid when splashing sounds may be heard. Palpation of the abdomen ventrally and to the right of the midline may indicate a tense area, impaction of the abomasum or enlarged reticulum and rumen, perhaps due to enzootic bovine leukosis. Deep palpation on the ventral left side of the rumen may indicate pain or discomfort in cases of traumatic reticulitis. Pinching the withers over the dorsal thoracic vertebrae can elicit pain and a reluctance to bend the back if done a second time. Deep palpation over the lower part of the ninth to eleventh ribs will produce a dull pain in omasal impaction. In calves abomasal distension can be determined by placing the hands under the right ventral abdomen and then lifting upwards two or three times.

Palpation of the left sublumbar fossa will indicate the frequency and intensity of ruminal contractions. Ruminal contractions reduce in indigestion or ruminal atony.

Percussion

Percussion can be carried out by drumming the fingers, or the use of a plexor or percussion hammer. When trying to detect the tinkling sounds of a displaced abomasum, flicking of the fingers is the best method. In normal cattle there is gas present in the rumen and so percussion of the left dorsal ruminal area will provide tympanic sounds but these decrease the more ventrally one investigates. The normal tympanitic sound becomes dull when there is ruminal impaction. There is an over-loud drum-like sound dorsally in ruminal tympany. Percussion of the left ventral abdomen will increase the tinkling sounds evident in left abomasal displacement. Likewise when used in the right lower flank sounds of right-sided displacement are heard.

Percussion and palpation will assist in the detection of fluid in the abdomen as with ascites, peritonitis with exudation, transudate of congestive heart failure.

Auscultation

On the left side are usually heard the roaring, gushing and grinding sounds of ruminal movement. The intensity of the sounds is lessened when contractions are reduced in their effectiveness. They are often decreased or absent in ruminal atony, ruminal tympany, traumatic peritonitis, left displacement of the abomasum, acute diffuse peritonitis. A tinkling sound is heard over the mid to lower third of the left side in left displacement of the abomasum. The sound is best heard 8–10 cm (3–4 in) along a line from the point of the elbow to the centre of the left sublumbar fossa. A widespread slight tinkle is heard in acute diffuse peritonitis in an otherwise noiseless abdomen.

On the right side the intestines produce gurgling and murmuring sounds and the large intestine is heard as a rumble and tinkling sound. Intestinal sounds become greater if peristalsis rate increases, as can happen with enteritis.

Auscultation of the trachea may allow detection of a grunt allied to reticular contractions in traumatic reticulitis.

Combined auscultation and percussion

This can be helpful in the detection in the abdomen of left side displacement of the abomasum, dilatation and torsion of the abomasum, caecal torsion and pneumoperitoneum. In the thorax fluid-filled intestine can be heard in diaphragmatic hernia.

Ballotment

The use of combined tactile palpation and percussion can be helpful in indicating the consistency of swelling. The fingers are quickly pushed into the area and kept in position. An organ underneath will be pushed away from the fingers and then return on to them. The technique is of use in detecting fluid and is very helpful in later pregnancy when used in the lower half of the right flank. Fluid in the abdomen is best detected by someone percussing on one side and then the fluid wave being detected on the other side.

Rectal examination

This is an essential part of the examination of the alimentary tract. When being undertaken there is sometimes a tendency for the rectum to balloon and make diagnosis difficult or impossible. In consequence it is best first to examine the organs as far cranially as possible. It should be possible to feel the left kidney and then to come backwards over the right kidney, reticulo-rumen and intestines. Diagnoses via the rectum are based on those given by Rosenberger (1977) (Figure 3.4).

1. Normal rectal palpation.
2. Vagal indigestion and distension of the rumen. Often the medial longitudinal groove between dorsal and ventral ruminal sacs is difficult to palpate and requires the rumen to be lifted.
3. Enlargement and torsion of the caecum which can be felt in the right dorsal area, occasionally the doughy form of the caecum can be felt in front of the pelvis. Mesenteric strands drawn to the left help indicate the torsion.
4. Right-sided enlargement and torsion of the abomasum. The abomasal surface resembles an inflated balloon. The attachment of the abomasal mucosal folds appears as parallel ridges.
5. Obstruction and enlargement of the abomasum. The organ will need to be lifted to be felt.
6. Enlarged abomasum displaced to the left. Usually this is not palpable per rectum. However the caudal edge of the greater omentum may be felt.
7. Intussusception of the small intestine. This is felt as a firm, fleshy spread of intestinal loop.
8. Torsion of the mesentery. The intestinal loops in the right half of the abdomen are enlarged and distended.

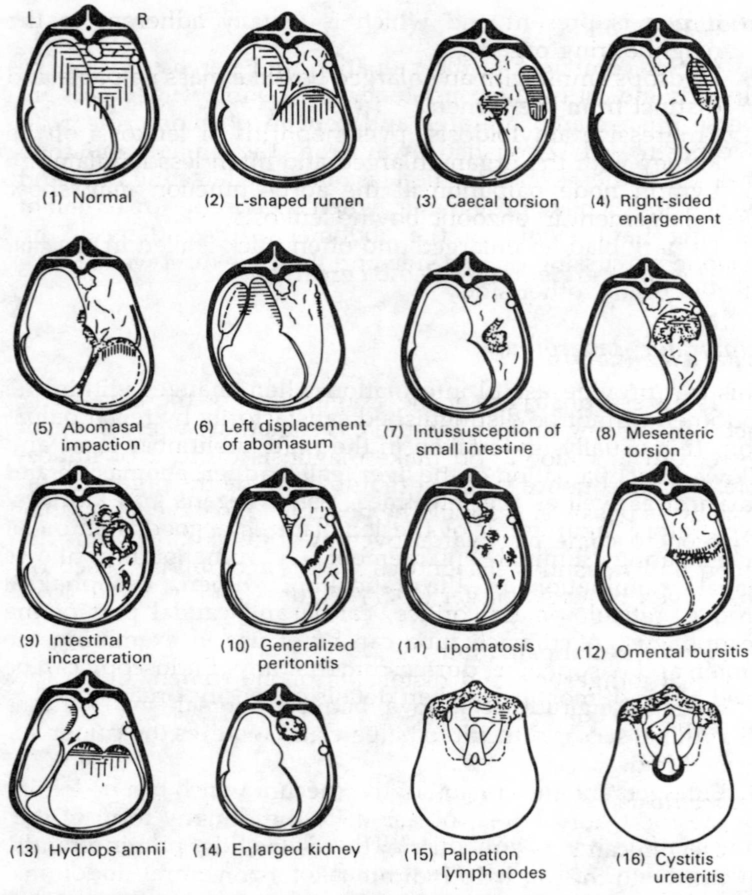

Figure 3.4 The main abnormalities detectable by palpation. The cross-section of the abdomen is viewed from behind. From Rosenberger *et al.* (1977), *Clinical examination of cattle*, 2nd edition (translated 1979 by R. Mack), Berlin, Verlag

9. Intestinal incarceration due to mesenteric rupture with herniation. The intestines feel firm and fleshy.
10. Generalized peritonitis felt as fibrinous or solid adhesions between kidneys and the rumen.
11. Fatty liver necrosis (lipomatosis) – one or more hard wax lumps are felt in the kidney fat, mesentery or elsewhere.
12. Omental bursitis extending to the pelvic inlet. One can feel a firm swelling running transversely which can be fluctuating

if pus is present and which is usually adherent to the neighbouring organs.

13. Hydrops amnii with an enlarged box-like mass palpable and distinct from the rumen.
14. Progressive amyloidosis, pyelonephritis or leukosis of the kidney with the organ enlarged and often less lobulated.
15. Lymph node palpation at the aortic junction may show enlargement in enzootic bovine leukosis.
16. Urinary bladder enlarged and often thick-walled in cystitis. The right ureters may also be enlarged.

Exploratory laparotomy

This can provide useful information when changes within the abdomen cannot be distinguished satisfactorily by rectal palpation. It is usually undertaken in the right sublumbar fossa and allows direct palpation of the liver, gall bladder, abomasum and omasum as well as the intestines, pelvic organs and kidneys. Exploratory laparotomy of the left flank is a good method of investigating ruminal enlargement. A rumenotomy allows visual examination of the reticulum, rumen, oesophageal groove, reticulo-omasal orifice, cardia and caudal part of the oesophagus. A stomach tube can be of use in examining the rumen and oesophagus during rumenotomy. Endoscopy can be used but is of most help when details of specific organs need to be seen.

Paracentesis

This is difficult in ruminant cattle because of the presence of the large rumen which takes up much of the ventral abdominal floor. When attempted care must be taken to keep this aseptic. A 5 cm (2 in) hypodermic needle of about 16 gauge is suitable. It can be placed to the left of the midline, 3–4 cm (1.5 in) medial and 5–7 cm (2–2.5 in) cranial to the foramen of the left subcutaneous abdominal vein. Another site of use is more cranial and situated just caudal to the xiphoid sternum and about 4–10 cm (2–4 in) lateral to the midline on the right side. Cattle will flinch as the abdominal muscles are penetrated and the peritoneum is entered. In normal adult animals about 1–5 ml of clear fluid is produced which will contain some mesothelial cells, lymphocytes, neutrophils and a few erythrocytes. Occasionally a few eosinophils and monocytes will be seen. The neutrophil:lymphocyte ratio is about 1:1.

Faecal examination

This obviously needs to be determined in terms of quantity, frequency of evacuation, nature, colour and odour.

Ruminal fluid examination

This can be helpful in determining the pH as well as protozoal numbers. These both tend to decrease in acidosis or caecal engorgement.

Metal detection

A metal detector will show the presence of metal within organs, usually the reticulorumen. If in a cranial part of the abdomen it may indicate a case of traumatic reticulitis. However metallic objects are found in the reticulorumen of many normal cattle.

Ruminal atony

When uncomplicated this is often referred to just as simple indigestion and is characterized by a lack of ruminal movements with a reduction in feed intake and reduced faecal output. It can be brought on by a great many different causes and can be a complication of other problems (Table 3.18). However most cases are of dietary or managemental origin and occur in dairy cattle, although ruminal atony does appear among beef cattle and calves. In severe ruminal atony there is acute rumen impaction.

Ruminal tympany

Perhaps better known as bloat, ruminal tympany is the overextension of the rumen with gas from fermentation. There are only two ways in which bloat can occur, firstly by interfering with normal reticuloruminal tone and motility and secondly by the partial or complete obstruction of the cardia preventing escape of gas from the rumen. Bloat is often designated as primary or secondary. Primary bloat (Table 3.19) is often considered to be frothy in nature and due to the type of feed offered, such as legumes. Secondary bloat (Table 3.20) is then defined as free gas and due to failure of eructation. The author does not personally support this type of classification as a large

Table 3.18 Some causes of ruminal atony

Dietary
Overfeeding of cereals (access to feed store; sudden, though often small, increase in concentrates; change in type of concentrates, change in person feeding, running out of concentrates after feeding *ad libitum* then feeding *ad libitum* again; running out of water, irregular feeding times, too infrequent feeding)
Change in type of cereal, e.g. oats to barley
Limited or irregular water supply
Depraved appetite causing ingestion of indigestible coarse material
Ingestion of large quantities of cold or frozen roughage
Sudden ingestion of large quantities of silage
Ingestion of poorly stored or spoiled feed

Therapy
Prolonged oral use of antibiotics or sulphonamides
Parenteral use of calcium salts
Overuse of formalin
Poor mixing of formalin
Use of anaesthetics
Use of central nervous system depressants
Use of prostaglandin

Other diseases
Abdominal pain
Abomasal dilatation/impaction torsion
Abomasal ulceration with perforation (chronic)
Acidosis
Alkalosis
Allergy
Cereal engorgement
Coliform mastitis (peracute)
Dehydration
Displaced abomasum
Hypocalcaemia
Intestinal dilatation
Pneumonia (acute bacterial)
Recumbency for whatever cause
Ruminal tympany
Traumatic reticulitis
Vagal indigestion

number of cases of gaseous bloat are the direct result of feeding, e.g. cereals.

There is another problem in that many bloats do not just contain gas but also some froth. Thus they are either semi-frothy or semi-gaseous. Even with frothy bloat, several factors are involved besides the food ingested. It is therefore possibly better to consider primary bloats to be those where the main sign is ruminal tympany due to feed, and secondary bloats to be those

Table 3.19 Some causes of primary bloat

Legume bloat (frothy)
  particularly clovers
  alteration in amount of saliva production
  alteration in constituents of saliva
  alteration in microorganisms present
  individual susceptibility

Cereal bloat (gaseous): often finely ground cereal
Abomasal bloat (gaseous): calves – usually bucket fed

Table 3.20 Some causes of secondary bloat

Abomasal ulceration
Actinobacillosis of oesophageal groove
Actinobacillosis of reticulum
Anaphylaxis
Botulism
Bovine viral diarrhoea (acute)
Choke
Cold water (ingestion)
Crude oil poisoning (some)
Diaphragmatic hernia (some cases)
Endocarditis
Enzootic bovine leukosis
Haemophilus somnus infection
Hormone weedkiller poisoning (calves)
Hydrocyanic acid poisoning
Hypersensitivity reaction
Hypoderma lineata larvae
Kale poisoning
Lacerations (infected) of oesophageal groove
Listeriosis
Lucerne feeding
Lymph node enlargement (posterior mediastinal in actinobacillosis, tuberculosis, *Actinomyces* (*Corynebacterium*) *pyogenes*
Lymphosarcoma (thymus)
Mucosal disease
Oesophageal lumen obstruction (pressure from mediastinal or bronchial lymph nodes)
Oesophageal obstruction
Oesophageal stricture
Oesophageal wall abscesses
Oesophagitis
Organophosphorus poisoning
Oxalate poisoning (acute)
Papillomatosis of oesophageal groove and reticulum
Parturient paresis (later stage postural change)
Rickets
Rumenitis

Table 3.20 continued

Ruminal atony
Sporadic bovine leukosis (thymic and generalized)
Tetanus
Traumatic peritonitis
Traumatic reticulitis
Tuberculosis (*Mycobacterium bovis*) – recurrent
Urea poisoning
Vagal indigestion (rumen hypermotility)
Vagal indigestion (ruminal atony)
Warble fly infestation
Water hemlock poisoning

due to some form of obstruction or alteration in normal ruminal function as well as the many other conditions in which bloat is a finding, although not necessarily a major one.

Abomasal dilatation

This is not a common condition in cattle but it does occasionally occur in calves (Table 3.21). It is usually due to obstruction of the pylorus.

Table 3.21 Some causes of abomasal dilatation

Physical
- Internal: hair balls, stones, acute intestinal obstruction, ingestion of coarse food (calves), abomasal ulceration
- External: lymphoma, fat necrosis

Abomasitis

Causes of inflammation of the abomasum are several and can be acute or chronic (Table 3.22).

Intestinal obstruction

This is not a common condition in cattle but can occur particularly in calves (Table 3.23). The most common type depends on the age of the animal. In adult cattle intussusception is most frequently seen, although in calves torsion of the mesentery is also often observed.

Table 3.22 Some causes of abomasitis

Physical
Gross overeating of cereal, eating frozen root crops, eating of fibrous bedding (chronic), eating mouldy or partially fermented feed, dental problems, paradontal disease, foreign bodies

Chemical
Irritants, e.g. arsenic, lead, copper, mercury, phosphorus
Excessive ruminal lactic acid production after cereal engorgement

Bacterial
Oral necrobacillosis in calves (*Fusiformis necrophorus*), colibacillosis (calves), enterotoxaemia (*Clostridium perfringens* (*welchii*) types A,B,C,D)

Viral
Mucosal disease, rinderpest, bovine malignant catarrh

Fungal
Mucor spp., *Aspergillus* spp.

Parasitic
Nematodes (*Trichostrongylus axei, Ostertagia ostertagi, Haemonchus contortus*)

Table 3.23 Some causes of intestinal obstruction

Physical
Caecal dilatation, caecal torsion
Herniation through mesentery
Herniation through ventral bladder ligament
Intussusception (common)
Mesenteric torsion (common in calves)

Alimentary dilatation

Table 3.24 Some causes of alimentary dilatation

Abdominal fat necrosis
Lipomas
Overfeeding cereal
Fibre balls

Enteritis

This encompasses a large number of different conditions but usually it is intestinal inflammation. Enteritis can be the result of infections due to bacteria, viruses, protozoal or metazoan parasites, chemical and physical causes. Other problems include deficiencies and indigestion. The end result is an interference with normal peristalsis and the production of diarrhoea and dysentery. There is a varying degree of dehydration and abdominal discomfort or pain is present in some cases.

Diarrhoea

Diarrhoea is a problem in many different conditions and is probably best dealt with by dividing it into the age of animal, i.e. calf (Table 3.25), growing animal (Table 3.26), or adult (Table 3.27). It should, however, be realized that not all cases of diarrhoea are the result of enteritis, but it can be due to other alimentary conditions as well as other organs such as the liver, kidneys or heart.

Peritonitis

This is a relatively uncommon condition in cattle (Table 3.28). It results in septicaemia or toxaemia, paralytic ileus, an accumulation of abdominal fluid and development of adhesions. Acute forms can be divided into acute diffuse or acute local. A chronic form is also seen.

Constipation

This occurs when the motility of the alimentary tract is reduced, thereby increasing the time for water absorption (Table 3.29). This results in the passage of small quantities of hard faeces. Tenesmus (see Table 3.30) may be apparent.

Tenesmus

This is usually the result of problems affecting the organs present within the pelvic cavity (Table 3.30). Although it can involve the alimentary tract, the urogenital system may be the site of the problem.

Table 3.25 Differential diagnosis of some of the causes of diarrhoea in calves

Condition	*Normal age when apparent*	*Frequency of occurrence*	*Epidemiology*	*Presence of blood*	*Attitude*	*Acute or chronic signs*	*Pyrexia*	*Diagnosis*
Mucosal disease	Any age	Rare	Non-immune dam	Occasionally	Dull	Both	Yes	Virus isolation serology
Clostridium perfringens (*welchii*) types B and C	10 days	Uncommon	Good condition calf	Yes	Dull	Acute	Yes	Faecal swab
Dietary scour	Up to 4 weeks	Very common	Management	No	Bright	Both	No	Faecal swab
Colibacillosis	Up to 1 week	Very common	Management/ colostrum	Occasionally	Dull	Acute	Early stages	Faecal swab
Rotavirus	About 1 week	Common	Overcrowding	No	Dull	Acute	Sometimes	Virus isolation serology
Adenovirus	About 1 week	? Rare	—	No	Dull	Acute	Slight	Virus isolation serology
Enterovirus	First few days	? Rare	Carrier cows	No	Dull	Acute	Yes	Serology
Infectious bovine rhinotracheitis (alimentary)	First few days	? Rare	Herd infection	No	Dull	Acute	Yes	Virus isolation serology
Astrovirus	? First few days	? Rare	Carrier cows	No	Dull	Acute	—	Virus isolation serology
Salmonella dublin	Over 2 weeks old	Common	Carrier cows	Often	Dull	Acute	Yes	Faecal swab
Other *Salmonella* infections	Over 2 weeks old	Common	Contaminated feed/water	Often	Dull	Acute	Yes	Faecal swab

Calicivirus	? First few days	? Rare	? Carrier cows	No	Dull	Acute	—	Virus isolation serology
Fringed particles	First few days	Very rare	? Carrier cows	No	Dull	Acute	—	Virus isolation
Coronavirus	Up to 3 weeks	Common	Overcrowding	No	Dull	Acute	Occasionally	Virus isolation
Campylobacter spp. infection	Over 1 week	Uncommon	Probably carriers	No	Slightly dull	Acute	Slight	Faecal swab
Proteus spp., *Pseudomonas* spp.	Over 10 days	Rare	Prolonged antibiotic usage	No	Slightly dull	Chronic	No	Faecal swab
Candida spp.	Over 10 days	Rare	Prolonged antibiotic usage	No	Slightly dull	Chronic	No	Faecal swab
Intestinal disaccharidase deficiency	From birth	Rare	Lack of enzyme	No	Slightly dull	Chronic	No	Glucose tolerance
Cryptosporidiosis	Over 10 days old	Common	Faecal spread	No	Slight dullness	Acute	No	Oocysts in faeces
Coccidiosis	Over 4 weeks	Common	Overcrowding, contaminated feed	Yes	Slightly dull	Subacute	Occasionally	Oocysts in faeces
Arsenic poisoning	Over 10 days	Very rare	Source of arsenic	Occasionally	Very dull	Peracute	No	Arsenic in urine, liver and kidney
Fluorosis	Over 4 weeks	Very rare	Source of fluoride	No	Dull	Acute	No	Blood and urine fluoride levels
Copper poisoning	Towards 3 months	Rare	Injection or pasture dressing	Some	Very dull	Both	Subnormal	Blood and liver copper levels
Sodium chloride poisoning	Over 5 weeks	Rare	Water supply interruption	No	Slight dullness	Acute	No	Blood sodium levels

Table 3.25 continued

Condition	*Normal age when apparent*	*Frequency of occurrence*	*Epidemiology*	*Presence of blood*	*Attitude*	*Acute or chronic signs*	*Pyrexia*	*Diagnosis*
Mercury poisoning	Over 10 days	Very rare	Seed grain used	Some	Dull	Both	No	Urine and kidney mercury levels
Molybdenum poisoning	Towards 3 months	Rare	Area of country	No	Some dullness	Both	No	Blood copper levels
Nitrate poisoning	Over 5 weeks	Uncommon	High nitrogen usage	No	Dull	Acute	No	Methaemoglobin
Aflatoxicosis	Towards 3 months	Rare	Groundnut usually	Occasionally	Dull	Acute	No	Feed analysis
Lead poisoning	Over 2 weeks	Uncommon	Batteries, paint, etc.	No	Excitable	Usually acute	Very slight	Blood and kidney lead levels
Tuberculosis	Any age	Very rare	Infected milk	No	Normal or slightly dull	Chronic	Slight	Tuberculin test
Furazolidone poisoning	Any age	Rare	Furazolidone previously in feed	Yes	Dull	Chronic	No	History of feeding furazolidone
Vitamin A deficiency	Any age	Rare	Lack of vitamin A and carotene	No	Dull but some have convulsions	Chronic	No	Plasma and liver vitamin A levels
Copper deficiency	3 months	Rare	Lack of copper	No	Some dullness	Chronic	No	Blood and kidney copper levels

From *Calf Management and Disease Notes*, A. H. Andrews, 1983, published by the Author, Welwyn.

Table 3.26 Differential diagnosis of some of the causes of diarrhoea in growing cattle

Condition	*Group or single problem*	*Frequency of occurrence*	*Epidemiology, history*	*Presence of blood*	*Attitude*	*Acute or chronic signs*	*Pyrexia*	*Diagnosis*
Acidosis	Group or single	Common	Access to excess carbohydrate	No	Dull	Acute	No	Signs, history
Actinobacillosis of reticulorumen	Single	Uncommon	Intermittent diarrhoea ± bloat	No	Normal	Chronic	No	History intermittent diarrhoea
Actinomycosis of reticulorumen	Single	Uncommon	Intermittent diarrhoea ± bloat	No	Normal	Chronic	No	History intermittent diarrhoea
Aflatoxicosis	Group	Uncommon	Diet	Yes	Dullness	Acute	No	Toxin detection
Amyloidosis	Single	Rare	Individual problem	No	Dull	Chronic	No	Signs, oedema
Anaphylaxis	Single	Uncommon	Injection; oral	No	Variable	Acute	Yes	History
Anthrax – acute	Single	Uncommon	Usually in feed	Sometimes	Dull	Acute	Yes	Signs, history
Antibiotic contamination of feed	Group	Uncommon	New batch of feed introduced	No	Dull	Acute	No	History, ketosis, recovery after feed removal
Arsenic poisoning (acute, subacute)	Group	Uncommon	Area	Yes	Dullness	Acute	No	Urine arsenic levels
Bacillary haemoglobinuria	Single	Rare	Good condition	Usually no	Dull	Acute	Yes	Signs, bacteriology
Bracken poisoning	Single/few	Uncommon	Usually young bracken	Yes	Dull	Acute	Yes	History, white cell, platelet, erythrocyte depression
Brassica spp. poisoning	Few	Not uncommon	Kale fed for several weeks	Usually no	Dull	Acute	Usually no	History, anaemia, Heinz–Ehrlich bodies
Bunostomiasis (subacute)	Group	Rare	Pasture	No	Variable	Subacute	No	Faecal egg count
Cobalt deficiency	Group	Not common	Area, heavy liming	No	Slight dullness	Chronic	No	Signs, history, plasma vitamin B_{12} levels
Coccidiosis	Group	Quite common	Overcrowding, poor hygiene	Yes	Dull	Acute/chronic	No	Oocysts in faeces
Copper deficiency	Group	Common	Area, molybdenum presence	No	Slight dullness	Chronic	No	Signs, history, plasma and liver copper

Table 3.26 continued

Condition	*Group or single problem*	*Frequency of occurrence*	*Epidemiology, history*	*Presence of blood*	*Attitude*	*Acute or chronic signs*	*Pyrexia*	*Diagnosis*
Copper poisoning (acute, chronic)	Single or group	Uncommon	Diet, injections	Yes	Dullness	Acute or chronic	No	Plasma copper levels
Dicrocoelium dendriticum infestation	Group	Uncommon	Pasture	No	Slight dullness	Chronic	No	Faecal egg count
Ergot poisoning	Single	Rare	Diet	No	Depression	Acute	No	Presence of ergots
Fascioliasis	Group	Not uncommon	Wet area where snail host survives	Yes (acute) No (chronic)	Dull	Acute/chronic	No	Faecal egg count
Fluorosis	Group	Uncommon	Diet, area	No	Variable	Acute	No	Blood fluorine levels
Haemonchosis (subacute) (diarrhoea uncommon)	Group	Quite common	Pasture	No	Slight dullness	Acute	No	Faecal egg count
Hypomagnesaemia	Group	Common	Diet, pasture, weather	No	Hyperaesthetic	Acute	Yes	Serum magnesium levels
Lead poisoning	Group	Common	Paint or other source of lead	Sometimes	Hyperexcitable	Acute	Usually	Kidney and liver lead levels
Linseed poisoning (acute)	Single or group	Rare	Diet	No	Dullness	Acute	No	Signs, history
Listeriosis (septicaemic)	Single/small group	Uncommon	Silage feeding	No	Depression	Acute	Yes	Signs, bacteriology, serology
Malignant catarrhal fever	Single	Uncommon	Often association with sheep, deer	Usually no	Depression	Acute	Yes	Signs
Mercury poisoning	Single or group	Rare	Diet	Yes	Hyperaesthesia	Acute and chronic	No	Signs, post mortem
Molybdenum poisoning	Group	Common	Area	No	Slight dullness	Chronic	No	Plasma copper levels

Monensin poisoning	Group	Rare	Overfeeding monensin	No	Dull	Acute	No	History
Mucosal disease	Single or group	Common	Usually over 6 months	Sometimes	Depression	Acute and chronic	Yes	Virus isolation, serology
Oak poisoning	Single/few	Rare	Acorns being eaten	Yes	Dull	Acute	No	History
Oesophagostomiasis	Group	Rare	Pasture	No	Variable	Subacute	No	Faecal egg count
Organophosphorus poisoning	Single	Rare	Use of organophosphorus compounds	No	Hyperexcitable	Acute	Some	History, blood cholinesterase levels
Parasitic bronchitis (unusual or early sign)	Group	Common	Pasture	No	Dull	Relatively acute	No	Faecal larval count
Parasitic gastroenteritis	Group	Common	Pasture grazed previously by infested animals	No	Dull later	Usually chronic	No	Faecal egg count
Ragwort poisoning	Few	Uncommon	Access, usually in hay	Usually no	Dull	Acute/chronic	No	History, liver biopsy
Redwater fever	Group	Common	Tick area	No	Slight dullness	Acute	Yes	Signs, organism present in blood
Salmonella dublin infection	Single	Common	Carrier animal	Often	Dull	Acute	Yes	Faecal swab, serum agglutination test
Salmonellosis	Single/group	Common	Contaminated feed or water	Often	Dull	Acute/chronic	Yes	Faecal swab, serum agglutination test
Selenium deficiency	Group	Not common	Area	No	Often normal	Chronic	No	Low glutathione peroxidase blood level
Sodium chloride poisoning	Single/group	Rare	Diet	No	Hyperaesthesia	Acute	No	Serum sodium levels
Tapeworm infestation	Group	Common but disease unusual	Pasture	Occasional	Bright	Chronic	No	Proglottides and eggs in faeces
Vitamin A deficiency	Group	Uncommon	Diet	No	Often normal	Chronic	No	Plasma vitamin A and carotene levels
Winter dysentery	Group	Common	Area problem	Yes	Slightly dull	Acute	Slight	History, bacteriology

From *Growing Cattle Management and Disease Notes*, Part 2 – Disease. A. H. Andrews, 1986, published by the Author, Welwyn.

Table 3.27 Differential diagnosis of some of the causes of diarrhoea in adult cattle

Condition	*Group or single problem*	*Frequency of occurrence*	*Epidemiology, history*	*Presence of blood*	*Attitude*	*Acute or chronic signs*	*Pyrexia*	*Diagnosis*
Acidosis	Group or single	Common	Access to excess carbohydrate	No	Dull	Acute	No	Signs, history
Actinobacillosis of reticulo-rumen	Single	Uncommon	Intermittent diarrhoea ± bloat	No	Normal	Chronic	No	History intermittent diarrhoea
Actinomycosis of reticulo-rumen	Single	Uncommon	Intermittent diarrhoea ± bloat	No	Normal	Chronic	No	History intermittent diarrhoea
Aflatoxicosis	Group	Uncommon	Diet	Yes	Dull	Acute	No	Toxin detection
Amyloidosis	Single	Rare	Individual problem	No	Dull	Chronic	No	Signs, oedema
Anaphylaxis	Single	Uncommon	Injection; oral	No	Variable	Acute	Yes	History
Anthrax – acute	Single	Uncommon	Usually in feed	Sometimes	Dull	Acute	Yes	Signs, history
Antibiotic contamination of feed	Group	Uncommon	New batch of feed introduced	No	Dull	Acute	No	History, ketosis, recovery after feed removal
Arsenic poisoning (acute, subacute)	Group	Uncommon	Area	Yes	Dull	Acute	No	Urine arsenic levels

Bacillary haemoglobinuria	Single	Rare	Good condition	Usually no	Dull	Acute	Yes	Signs, bacteriology
Bracken poisoning	Single/few	Uncommon	Usually young bracken	Yes	Dull	Acute	Yes	History, white cell, platelet, erythrocyte depression
Brassica spp. poisoning	Few	Not uncommon	Kale fed for several weeks	Usually no	Dull	Acute	Usually no	History, anaemia, Heinz–Ehrlich bodies
Bunostomiasis (subacute)	Group	Rare	Pasture	No	Variable	Subacute	No	Faecal egg count
Cobalt deficiency	Group	Not common	Area, heavy liming	No	Slight dullness	Chronic	No	Signs, history, plasma B_{12} levels
Congestive heart failure	Single	Uncommon	Long-standing dyspnoea, oedema	No	Dull	Chronic	No	Signs; murmur, oedema
Copper deficiency	Group	Common	Area, molybdenum presence	No	Slight dullness	Chronic	No	Signs, history, plasma and liver copper
Copper poisoning (acute, chronic)	Single or group	Uncommon	Diet, injections	Yes	Dullness	Acute or chronic	No	Plasma copper levels
Dicrocoelium dendriticum infestation	Group	Uncommon	Pasture	No	Slight dullness	Chronic	No	Faecal egg count
Ergot poisoning	Single	Rare	Diet	No	Depression	Acute	No	Presence of ergot

Table 3.27 continued

Condition	*Group or single problem*	*Frequency of occurrence*	*Epidemiology, history*	*Presence of blood*	*Attitude*	*Acute or chronic signs*	*Pyrexia*	*Diagnosis*
Fascioliasis	Group	Uncommon	Wet area where snail host survives	Yes (acute) No (chronic)	Dull	Acute or chronic	No	Faecal egg count
Fluorosis	Group	Uncommon	Diet, area	No	Variable	Acute	No	Blood fluorine levels
Grass (scour)	Group	Common	Usually spring or heavily fertilized	No	Normal	Acute	No	History
Haemonchosis (subacute) [diarrhoea uncommon]	Group	Quite common	Pasture	No	Slight dullness	Acute	No	Faecal egg count
Hypomagnesaemia	Group	Common	Diet, pasture, weather	No	Hyperaesthetic	Acute	Yes	Serum magnesium levels
Johne's disease	Group but usually signs in one	Quite common	Herd history	No	Bright	Chronic	No	Presence of acid-fast organisms, CFT
Lead poisoning	Group	Common	Paint or other source of lead	Sometimes	Hyperexcitable	Acute	Usually	Kidney and liver lead levels
Linseed poisoning (acute)	Single or group	Rare	Diet	No	Dullness	Acute	No	Signs, history

Listeriosis (septicaemic)	Single or small group	Uncommon	Silage feeding	No	Depression	Acute	Yes	Signs, serology, bacteriology
Malignant catarrhal fever	Single	Uncommon	Often association with sheep, deer	Usually no	Depression	Acute	Yes	Signs
Mercury poisoning	Single or group	Rare	Diet	Yes	Hyperaesthesia	Acute and chronic	No	Signs, post mortem
Molybdenum poisoning	Group	Common	Area	No	Slight dullness	Chronic	No	Plasma copper levels
Monensin poisoning	Group	Rare	Overfeeding monensin	No	Dull	Acute	No	History
Mucosal disease	Single or group	Common	Usually over 6 months	Sometimes	Depression	Acute and chronic	Yes	Virus isolation, serology
Nitrite poisoning	Usually group	Uncommon	Poor animal, bad spreading fertilizer, rotting plant matter	No	Dull	Acute	No	Signs, methaemoglobinaemia
Oak poisoning	Single/few	Rare	Acorns being eaten	Yes	Dull	Acute	No	History
Oesophagostomiasis	Group	Rare	Pasture	No	Variable	Subacute	No	Faecal egg count
Organophosphorus poisoning	Single	Rare	Use of organophosphorus compounds	No	Hyperexcitable	Acute	Some	History, blood cholinesterase levels
Paradontal disease	Single	Uncommon to see signs	Old, loose teeth, quidding, saliva drooling	No	Usually normal	Chronic	No	Signs

Table 3.27 continued

Condition	*Group or single problem*	*Frequency of occurrence*	*Epidemiology, history*	*Presence of blood*	*Attitude*	*Acute or chronic signs*	*Pyrexia*	*Diagnosis*
Parasitic bronchitis (unusual or early signs)	Group	Common	Pasture	No	Dull	Relatively acute	No	Faecal larval count
Parasitic gastroenteritis	Group	Very uncommon. Usually exposed previously	Pasture grazed previously by infested animals	No	Dull later	Usually chronic	No	Faecal egg count
Phosphorus poisoning (acute, subacute)	Group	Very uncommon	Access to phosphorus, abdominal pain	No	Dull	Acute	No	Signs, access to phosphorus
Ragwort poisoning	Few	Uncommon	Access, usually in hay	Usually no	Dull	Acute or chronic	No	History, liver biopsy
Redwater fever	Group	Common	Tick area	No	Slight dullness	Acute	Yes	Signs, organism present
Salmonella dublin infection	Single	Common	Carrier animal	Often	Dull	Acute	Yes	Faecal swab, serum agglutination test
Salmonellosis	Single or group	Common	Contaminated feed or water	Often	Dull	Acute or chronic	Yes	Faecal swab, serum agglutination test
Selenium deficiency	Group	Not common	Area	No	Often normal	Chronic	No	Low glutathione peroxidase levels

Silage (chronic)	Group	Common	Butyric silage	No	Dull	Variable	No	Silage analysis
Sodium chloride poisoning	Single or group	Rare	Diet	No	Hyperaesthesia	Acute	No	Serum sodium levels
Tapeworm infestation	Group	Common but disease unusual	Pasture	Occasional	Bright	Chronic	No	Proglottides and eggs in faeces
Upper alimentary squamous cell carcinoma (diarrhoea and wasting syndrome)	Single	Not common	Old cow, bracken area	No	Dull	Chronic	No	Area, oral papillomas
Winter dysentery	Group	Common	Area problem	Yes	Slightly dull	Acute	Slight	History, bacteriology

From *Adult Cattle Management and Disease Notes* (not yet published). A. H. Andrews, Welwyn.

Table 3.28 Some causes of peritonitis

Abdominal wall perforation (trauma)
Abomasal torsion
Abomasal ulcer perforation
Abscess rupture
Actinomycosis
Enzootic bovine leukosis
Hepatic abscess
Laparotomy
Rumenitis, acute
Rumenotomy
Splenic abscess
Traumatic reticulitis
Tuberculosis
Umbilical vessel abscess
Uterine catheterization (inexpert)
Uterine rupture
Vaginal rupture (coitus or sadistic)

Table 3.29 Some causes of constipation

Abomasal impaction (some)
Acetonaemia (not real consequence)
Bacillary haemoglobinuria
Botulism (some cases)
Displaced abomasum (right-sided – some)
Endocarditis
Fever
Fluorosis (acute, some cases)
Haemonchosis
Hepatitis
Indigestion (simple) – scanty, dry faeces
Liver abscess necrobacillosis (chronic)
Oak poisoning
Oesophagostomiasis (early signs)
Omasal impaction (slight)
Parturient paresis
Redwater fever
Ruminal atony – scanty, dry faeces
Septicaemia
Tapeworm infestation
Tetanus
Toxaemia
Traumatic pericarditis (some)
Traumatic reticulitis
Zinc poisoning

Table 3.30 Some causes of excessive straining (tenesmus)

Abortion
Aflatoxicosis
Bovine viral diarrhoea
Cervicitis
Coccidiosis
Constipation
Contagious pyelonephritis
Cystitis
Diarrhoea
Intussusception
Mucosal disease
Parturition
Placental retention
Rabies
Ragwort poisoning
Rinderpest
Salmonella (acute enteritis)
Urethral calculi
Urethritis
Vaginitis

Table 3.31 Some causes of acute colic

Abomasal dilatation (acute)
Abomasal torsion
Arsenic poisoning
Clostridium perfringens types A, B, C, D, E
Contagious bovine pleuropneumonia (some cases)
Copper poisoning (acute)
Hemlock poisoning
Intestinal obstruction (acute)
Lead poisoning
Nitrate/nitrite poisoning
Oak poisoning
Phosphorus poisoning
Renal calculi (pelvis blockage)
Rhododendron poisoning
Rinderpest (later stages)
Salmonellosis
Selenium poisoning
Sodium chloride poisoning
Sulphur poisoning
Urea poisoning

Colic

Abdominal pain resulting in characteristically observable signs as with the horse is much less common in cattle. Signs similar to the horse do occur in acute colic (Table 3.31) with bouts of severe discomfort, restlessness, kicking and constantly going down and rising.

Causes of subacute and mild colic are given in Tables 3.32 and 3.33 respectively.

Table 3.32 Some causes of subacute colic

Cystitis (when acute)
Hepatitis (some cases)
Monochloroacetate poisoning
Omasal atony (acute)
Oxalate poisoning (acute)
Pericarditis
Peritonitis – acute diffuse
Ragwort poisoning
Traumatic reticulitis
Urethral calculi

Table 3.33 Some causes of mild colic

Abomasal dilatation (chronic)
Abomasal impaction
Abomasal ulceration
Abomasitis – acute
Abomasitis – chronic (some)
Caecal dilatation
Caecal torsion
Cereal engorgement (mild form)
Diaphragmatic hernia (severe form)
Displaced abomasum (left)
Lipomatosis (intermittent)
Liver abscess necrobacillosis (acute)
Omasal impaction
Peritonitis, acute diffuse
Peritonitis, chronic (intermittent signs)
Ruminal tympany
Silage feeding (sudden gross ingestion resulting in indigestion)

4 Liver

External palpation
Liver biopsy
Laboratory testing
Jaundice
Hepatitis

The liver is one of the most important organs of the animal; without it death ensues, hence the name. In cattle, as in all other animals, it has a diversity of roles and is involved in many forms of disease. It is thus unfortunate that any assessment of hepatic status is difficult. Fortunately primary problems of the liver, other than perhaps fatty liver and fascioliasis, are rare. However, secondary conditions with liver involvement are common. When problems do occur it often means that much of the large reserve of hepatic tissue has been damaged and in many instances, once signs are apparent, the condition is irreversible.

The liver has many functions, including:

1. Secretion of bile.
2. Formation and storage of glycogen and regulation of glucose level in blood. Gluconeogenesis is undertaken and if failure occurs it results in lower circulating glucose levels and raised ketone levels. Fatty liver can also result.
3. Deamination of amino acids and urea formation.
4. Destruction of uric acid.
5. Synthesis of fatty acids from carbohydrate and protein, phosphorylation of fats, the interaction of fatty acids, partial oxidation of fatty acids, ketone body formation.
6. Storage of vitamin A.
7. Detoxification of toxic sulphur transported to it in the blood.
8. Helping to destroy erythrocytes.
9. Storage and stimulation of antipernicious anaemia factor.
10. Formation of fibrinogen and albumin as well as other plasma proteins.
11. Formation of prothrombin.
12. Destruction of oestrogens.

External palpation

It is not possible to palpate the liver externally in the normal animal as it is enclosed within the costal arch. Occasionally if it is grossly enlarged it can be felt in the right sublumbar fossa.

Liver biopsy

This is a very useful technique to determine the structure of the liver, provided any problem present within it is diffuse. Unfortunately it does rely on histological examination and so often it is some time before a result is obtained. Various methods of staining liver biopsies are available and in the past a biopsy needle has been used with a syringe. The author prefers the use of a 'Tru-Cut' biopsy needle (Travenol Laboratories, Thetford) which, although expensive, does seem to result in few problems in the patient. The technique used is to wash over the biopsy site well, after insertion of a small amount of local anaesthetic. The animal should be restrained in a crush. The site is in the eleventh rib intercostal space at about the level of a line drawn from the mid-point of the right sublumbar fossa. At this point no lung will be encountered in the normal animal (Figure 4.1). The needle is placed through the skin incision and directed cranially and ventrally for about 7.5 cm (3 in). The biopsy is then taken and if necessary further samples can be obtained.

The test will indicate generalized liver problems as well as conditions such as fatty liver when over 20% of the hepatic tissue consists of fat.

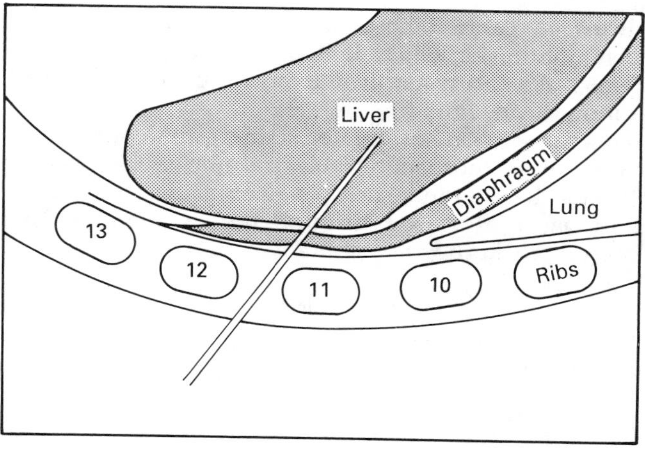

Figure 4.1 Diagrammatic frontal view showing relationship of the liver, ribs and lungs when taking a liver biopsy. After Pearson, E. G. and Craig, A. M. (1980), *Modern Veterinary Practice*, **61**, 237

Laboratory testing

Laboratory tests often have to be used to determine function or possible disease. No tests are completely specific; however several are used.

1. Haematology: white cell count or differential levels are of little use.
   Erythrocyte level can be helpful and anaemia occurs in some chronic conditions.

2. Blood protein levels: the liver produces albumin and so low levels possibly indicate a chronic problem, although they can be due to poor protein intake by the animal, protein leakage or poor digestibility and uptake of amino acids as well as some kidney problems. When due to liver problems, albumin reduction is a result of several weeks' malnutrition before signs occur. Haemoglobin levels also fall and if there is lowered haemoglobin and albumin but a normal globulin level it is quite likely to be the result of hepatic dysfunction. Raised serum globulin levels can occur if there is an infection or autoimmune disease is present affecting the liver or other organs.

Jaundice

Jaundice (see Table 2.42) is not a common finding in cattle. When it occurs, however, it is usually a clinical sign of liver problems but it can result from overproduction of bile salts, e.g. in haemolytic anaemia (Figure 4.2).

Direct bilirubin causes greater staining than indirect, there is therefore much more noticeable staining with obstructive or hepatic cell degeneration than in haemolytic anaemia. Indirect bilirubin has not passed through the liver and so it is not possible for the kidney to excrete it. Thus in haemolytic disease

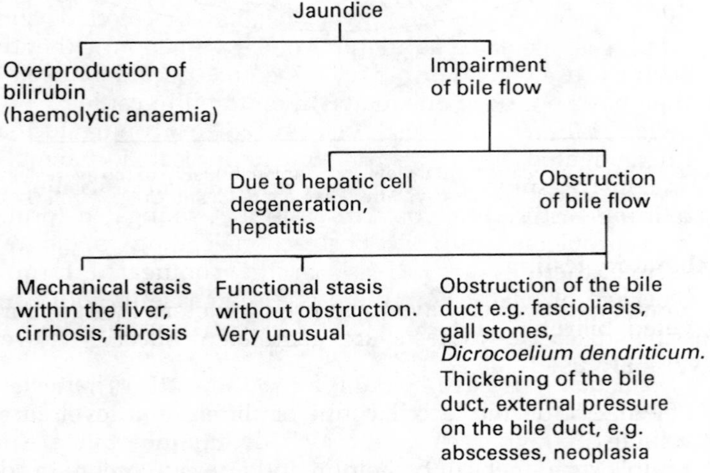

Figure 4.2 Some causes of jaundice in cattle

there are high quantities of indirect bilirubin in the serum and urobilinogen in the urine is increased but there is no bilirubin present in the latter.

In cases of bile obstruction there is usually a more severe jaundice and in many cases bile salts are absent from the faeces. There is an increase in direct bilirubin in the circulation and this can be excreted by the kidney and results in high levels within the urine. Urobilinogen and indirect bilirubin may also be present in the blood. The amount of urobilinogen present depends on whether bilirubin reaches the intestine and is converted to urobilinogen and then reabsorbed.

Liver function tests

1. *Bromosulphophthalein test (BSP)* can be undertaken in cattle. This involves injecting the dye intravenously and taking samples at intervals. There is some variation in the results in cattle and it is often best to test a suspect animal and a control together. A few normal cattle have still had some dye present after 30 minutes but this is unusual. In cattle with liver dysfunction the dye is retained for 45 minutes or longer. The test is time-consuming but does indicate recent damage. It is the best functional test presently available for cattle and samples should be taken at 5 and 9 minutes after injection. The serum is made alkaline and the dye quantity measured by a spectrophotometer. The results are plotted and a half-life is calculated as an index of liver function. Other dyes such as rose bengal or indocyanine green could be used but they have not been adequately monitored in cattle.
2. *Serum bilirubin* has also been used in conjugated and unconjugated form. As previously indicated, haemolytic anaemia results mainly in an increase in unconjugated bilirubin with a limited increase in the conjugated form. In liver problems with bile obstruction leading to failure to secrete there is an increase in the conjugated form. In blockage of biliary flow there is an increase in both conjugated bilirubin and, to a lesser extent, unconjugated bilirubin.
3. *Flocculation tests* have been little used in cattle. The tests are dependent on the fact that some colloidal solutes are more soluble in higher concentrations of albumin but are less soluble in higher concentrations of globulin and so tend to precipitate. Thus a decrease in albumin:globulin ratio results

in more precipitation. The tests are too insensitive and not specific to liver disease. Serum electrophoresis is probably of more use than the flocculation tests because it differentiates the individual serum protein classes.

4. *Increased serum enzyme activity* is often the first indication of hepatic disease.

   AST (aspartate aminotransferase), also known as SGOT (serum glutamine oxaloacetate transaminase) occurs in the case of organ or muscle damage where, in the latter case, the levels are often very high. It is not specific for liver problems but does rise in acute hepatic disease and also sometimes in more chronic problems.

   SAP (alkaline phosphatase) also rises in conditions involving other organs. It does tend to be high in severe obstruction of the bile ducts and biliary hyperplasia, hepatitis, cirrhosis or accumulation and deposition of fat. It is a relatively stable enzyme.

   ALT (L-alanine aminotransferase), also known as serum glutamine pyruvic transferase (SGPT) is of little use because there are only low concentrations of ALT in hepatic cells of ruminants and the enzyme is not very stable.

   SDH (sorbitol dehydrogenase) is a liver-specific enzyme mainly increased in cases of acute hepatic cell breakdown. It is an enzyme indicating current damage and it may not remain high throughout the course of a disease. It is not very stable at room temperature.

   LDH (lactic dehydrogenase) is concerned with catalysing the reaction of pyruvate to lactate and is found in many tissues. There are five different isoenzymes of LDH and a rise in serum levels of specific isoenzymes is more important than the total enzyme activity level. However, qualification of the enzymes is time-consuming and costlier than a total LDH analysis.

   GLDH (glutamate dehydrogenase) is concerned with cellular respiration. It is an enzyme specific to the liver and is found in the mitochondrial matrix of hepatocytes. It is highest in cells near the portal areas and also in the brain. Serum levels increase in liver damage and fascioliasis but not usually in non-hepatic disease. The enzyme is relatively specific and is fairly stable at room temperature.

   γGT (gamma glutamyltransferase) is a good indicator of bile duct damage. It is useful in chronic fascioliasis involving the bile ducts and so is relatively selective for cirrhosis. Massive fatty change can also result in raised γGT levels.

Bilirubin levels can be measured and again are an indicator of problems (see jaundice) but they are not always due to liver dysfunction.

5. *Propionate conversion test:* the liver is the main site of gluconeogenesis and propionate metabolism in ruminants of the volatile fatty acids (acetic, butyric, propionic). The test is gluconeogenic. Thus the measurement of glucose production after the intravenous injection of sodium propionate is useful in assessing the liver's ability for metabolic conversion.
6. *Exploratory laparotomy* can be of use by making an incision just caudal to the last rib in the right sublumbar fossa. It allows some visualization of the organ as well as palpation and will also enable a biopsy to be undertaken.
7. *Ultrasound* is a technique frequently undertaken for fertility investigations. It is likely to be of increasing use in liver examination.
8. *Paracentesis* has previously been discussed (see p. 75) and the same procedure is used. It can be of use if a liver condition is suspected. An abdominal transudate suggests liver disease

Table 4.1 Some causes of hepatitis

Infections
- Bacillary haemoglobinuria
- Leptospirosis
- Listeriosis
- Salmonellosis

Parasites
- Massive *Fasciola* infestation

Other conditions
- Congestive heart failure

Toxins
- Many poisonings
- Aflatoxins (*Aspergillus* spp. or algae)
- Arsenic
- Carbon tetrachloride
- Chloroform
- Coal tar
- Heliotrope (*Heliotropum europaeum*)
- Hexachloroethane
- *Penicillium rubrum*
- Phosphorus
- Ragwort (*Senecio jacobea*)
- Selenium

whereas a large amount of foul-smelling thin pus suggests diffuse peritonitis. This might be due to many different causes, including a ruptured hepatic abscess.

Hepatitis

As previously stated, the liver is involved in many different problems affecting the body. However, specific conditions resulting in hepatitis (Table 4.1) tend to be diagnosed relatively infrequently.

5 Cardiovascular system

Inspection
Palpation
Percussion
Auscultation
Abnormal sounds
Myocardial weakness
Endocarditis
Anaemia
Oedema

Heart

The heart is found in the chest and its base is between the third and sixth ribs. Its apex is roughly median in position, opposite the articulation of the sternum with the sixth costal cartilage and about 2 cm (1 in) cranial to the diaphragm. On the left side the heart is in contact with the thoracic wall between the third rib and the fourth intercostal space. On the right side there is less contact and it involves only a small area of the ventral part of the fourth rib and adjacent parts of the third and fourth intercostal spaces. The caudal border of the heart is dorsoventral and in contact with the pericardium. It is located opposite the fifth intercostal space. The right atrioventricular orifice is found on the fourth rib about 10 cm (4 in) above the costochondral junction. The pulmonary orifice is cranial to the atrioventricular orifice opposite the third intercostal space and higher. The left atrioventricular orifice is opposite the fourth intercostal space and the aortic orifice is alongside the fourth rib and about 12.5 cm (5 in) above the ventral sternal border.

When the ventricles are relaxing the atria tend to fill on the right from the cranial and caudal venae cavae and on the left from the pulmonary veins. When the atria contract blood is forced into the ventricles. When the latter have filled, they contract with closure of the atrioventricular valves and the tensing of the chordae tendineae. The first heart sound, often referred to as 'lub' or systolic sound, is due to ventricular contraction and corresponding valves. The effect is to force blood via the pulmonary artery into the lungs and, via the aorta, oxygenated blood to the body. As the ventricular contraction starts to end the atria relax and fill with blood from the veins. Then the ventricles start to relax, the circulatory blood pressure is reduced and this results in closure of the aortic and pulmonary valves. The closure of the valves results in the second heart sound, the 'dup' or diastolic sound. Thus the first sound of the heart corresponds to the start of ventricular systole and the second sound to the start of ventricular diastole. It is possible to hear a third sound following the normal beats and this is due to atrial contraction.

Cardiac examination

This is the most important part of the examination of the circulatory system.

Inspection

This is of very limited value as the organ has little contact with the chest wall. Signs of cardiac activity are thus considered to be abnormal unless the animal is very thin. If there is gross cardiac enlargement a larger area will be in contact with the chest wall. This in turn may be observable on the left and/or right sides.

Palpation

This gives an impression of the force of the cardiac beat. The pulse can be felt over the fourth left intercostal space and fifth rib. On the right side it is felt in a small area of the fourth intercostal space and fifth rib. There may appear to be more contact between the heart and chest wall.

Percussion

As with palpation, the area which can be percussed is small because of the surrounding tissues and thoracic cage (Figure 5.1). Percussion is thus mainly of value where there is an increase in cardiac area. The percussion area in the normal heart is small and over the left third and fourth intercostal spaces. The examination is aided by drawing forward the left front leg. It is of little use where animals have a thick chest wall or are fat. Percussion can indicate an increase in the area of cardiac dullness and this can be due to increase in size of the pericardial sac or the heart itself.

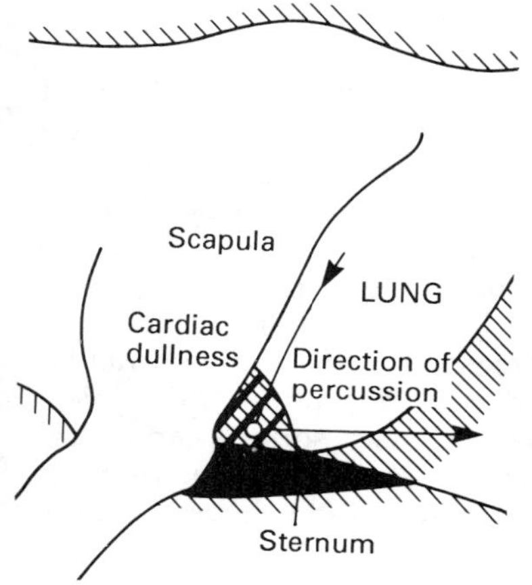

Figure 5.1 Percussion of the heart. Percussion should commence by moving ventrally in the area caudal to the scapula. Examination should continue by moving caudally from the area of cardiac dullness (after Kelley, W. R. (1967), *Veterinary Clinical Diagnosis*, London, Baillière Tindall and Cassell, p.98)

Auscultation

Obviously this is the main method for examining the heart. The first aim is to define the routine amplitude or intensity of the heart sounds, their rhythm, character or quality and their number or frequency as well as the presence of abnormal heart sounds. The second aim is to determine abnormal sounds either associated with or arising from the heart beat.

Volume

An increase in heart sounds is heard where there is greater muscular activity such as in cardiac hypertrophy. It also occurs in anaemia, lung consolidation and hypomagnesaemia. A reduction in volume occurs when the heart is weakened and this can be the result of pyrexia, septicaemia or toxaemia. It can also be caused by cardiac failure. If there is fluid in the pericardial sac the sounds may appear to be muffled.

Rhythm

In cattle, the rhythm of the heart is regular. However in abnormal animals the heart rate may be irregular or intermittent. When the heart rate exceeds about 90 beats/min the heart sounds tend to merge or blend. It can occasionally occur in normal cattle but will be lost on exercise. In cases of incomplete heart block the ventricles fail to respond to atrial contractions and so there are periods with no palpable pulse and no normal heart sounds. This is rare in cattle.

Character

The quality of the heart sounds can be compared. The volume of the first sound is related to the force of ventricular contraction and the second depends on the pressure in the great vessels at the time of ventricular diastole. If there is pulmonary obstruction so that an increase occurs in the pressure within the pulmonary arteries, then the volume of the sound produced by the pulmonary valves contracting is increased. In some cases there will also be a need to increase the force of ventricular contraction to allow entry of blood into the pulmonary arteries.

Reduplication of the first and second heart sounds can occur. In cases involving the first sound then it can occur when animals are healthy but have a high blood pressure and is heard in some normal cattle.

Frequency

Heart rate is usually similar to the pulse and variations have been dealt with under the latter (see p. 40). However, a weak heart can lead to a pulse deficit as the contractions fail to produce palpable pulse waves. Reduplication of the second sound can occur most frequently when there is an increase in pressure in the pulmonary artery.

Abnormal sounds

These may replace one or both the heart sounds or may be additional to them. Abnormal sounds or bruits occur in cardiac disease. Sounds can be endocardial or pericardial.

Endocardial

These are murmurs or bruits (Table 5.1) and are mainly associated with valvular problems. Occasionally they can be due to functional problems which interfere with the free flow of blood through the heart. The location of the murmur can be determined in relation to the heart cycle as presystolic, systolic or diastolic. They can vary in character so that a murmur due to stenosis tends to be rough, harsh and ragged, that due to regurgitation is softer and more like a purr and if tumultuous, as

Table 5.1 Some causes of heart sounds (murmur)

Anaemia
Cardiac defects – congenital (calf)
Coarctation of the aorta (systolic)
Diaphragmatic hernia (systolic)
Downer cow
Endocarditis (systolic or diastolic)
Enzootic bovine leukosis (cardiac form – systolic)
Myocardial weakness
Oesophageal obstruction (systolic)
Patent ductus arteriosus (calf – machinery murmur)
Ruminal tympany (systolic)
Tetanus (systolic)
Tetralogy of Fallot (calf)
Thrombosis of vena cava
Toxaemia
Vagal indigestion (systolic – rumen hypermotility)
Valvular disease
Ventricular septal defects (calf)

happens in anaemia, it can have a humming character. It may be possible to suggest the likely site by the area in which the sounds appear loudest.

Presystolic murmur

This occurs before the first heart sound (brr-lub-dup). It can indicate stenosis of the tricuspid (right atrioventricular) or mitral (left atrioventricular) valve.

Systolic murmur

This occurs between the heart sounds (lub-brr-dup) and can be due to tricuspid valve incompetence, mitral valve incompetence, pulmonary stenosis or aortic stenosis.

Diastolic murmur

This follows the second sound (lub-dup-brr) and the adventitious sound immediately follows the second heart sound. Aortic incompetence or possibly pulmonary valve incompetence may cause it.

Murmurs have been graded according to their intensity:

Grade I Just audible murmur only detectable after careful auscultation.

Grade II Faint murmur but clearly detectable after a few seconds' auscultation.

Grade III Murmur immediately audible on auscultation over a wide area.

Grade IV Very loud murmur accompanied by a thrill. It is not heard if only light pressure applied to sternum.

Grade V Extremely loud murmur with a thrill. It can be heard with only very light pressure of the stethoscope.

Pericardial

These sounds are relatively common in cattle and muffle or decrease the heart sounds. In the early stages they are rasping or rubbing sounds but later they become gurgling, tinkling or splashing sounds.

Electrocardiogram

Although it would be possible to do this in cattle it is rarely undertaken and will not be considered further.

Angiocardiogram

This is also possible but is not undertaken for economic reasons.

Paracentesis

This is occasionally performed to show pericarditis with septic exudate.

Myocardial weakness or asthenia

Conditions affecting the cardiac muscle in cattle are rare (Table 5.2). When they do occur they can result in a reduction in the cardiac reserve as well as acute heart failure or congestive heart failure.

Table 5.2 Some causes of myocardial weakness

Infections
Clostridium chauvoei infection (blackleg)
Foot-and-mouth disease
Enzootic bovine leukosis
Septicaemias
Nutritional
Copper deficiency (chronic)
Selenium deficiency
Vitamin E deficiency
Poisoning
Arsenic
Cotton seed
Mercury
Phosphorus
Selenium

Valvular disease

This is uncommon in cattle and can be congenital, which is rare, or acquired. The most frequently acquired form is that of endocarditis. The acquired valvular lesion most often seen is insufficiency of the right atrioventricular valve, followed by insufficiency of the left atrioventricular valve.

Endocarditis

This usually involves the valves and results in cardiac murmurs. Most cases of infection are bacterial in origin (Table 5.3). Many follow a septic focus in another organ or part of the body.

Table 5.3 Some causes of endocarditis

Bacterial
Actinomyces (Corynebacterium) pyogenes (often after nephritis, metritis, mastitis, traumatic reticulitis)
Clostridium chauvoei (blackleg)
Escherichia coli
Mycoplasma mycoides infection (contagious bovine pleuropneumonia)
Streptococci, alpha-haemolytic

Anaemia (Table 5.4)

Anaemia is a reduction in the oxygen-carrying capacity of the blood, either as a result of a decrease in red blood cells or the amount of haemoglobin present per unit volume of blood. It results in pale mucous membranes (see Table 2.39). There are

Table 5.4 Some causes of anaemia

Cobalt deficiency
Coccidiosis (chronic)
Copper deficiency
Enzootic haematuria
Enzootic bovine leukosis
Fascioliasis
Haemorrhage
Haemothorax
Iron deficiency (cows)
Leptospirosis
Lice infestation (sucking)
Molybdenosis
Oesophagostomiasis
Ostertagia type II
Oxalate poisoning (chronic)
Potassium deficiency
Pyridoxine deficiency
Redwater fever
Sarcosporidiosis
Thrombosis of vena cava
Water intoxication

many causes of the problem – haemorrhage, haemolysis or dyshaemopoiesis. Although haemorrhagic anaemia can be due to obvious haemorrhage, in other cases it may be a much more chronic problem as with parasitic disease. Usually signs are the result of an excessive breakdown of circulatory erythrocytes and can be either infectious or non-infectious. It can occur very suddenly although other cases will be more chronic in nature. Thus it is of value to look at the causes of haemoglobinaemia (see p.135). Dyshaemopoiesis is probably the largest category of disorders and it includes the failure of the bone marrow to produce enough red cells to monitor normal circulating numbers of erythrocytes.

Oedema (Table 5.5)

Oedema is the accumulation of fluid in tissue spaces. Fluid continually perfuses the tissues but when there is a disturbance in the mechanisms there is an alteration in the interchange between the capillaries, the tissues and the lymphatic vessels.

Table 5.5 Some causes of gross oedema

Amyloidosis (generalized)
Anaphylaxis
Bacillary haemoglobinuria (brisket)
Bee stings
Congestive heart failure (ascites, anasarca, hydrothorax, hydropericardium – right)
Contagious bovine pleuropneumonia (throat)
Copper poisoning (acute)
Endocarditis
Enzootic bovine leukosis – cardiac form (brisket and submandibular space)
Fascioliasis (submandibular)
Haemonchosis (submandibular, ventral, abdomen)
Haemorrhage (chronic)
Hypersensitivity reaction
Inherited lymphatic obstruction
Johne's disease (submandibular)
Lymph node enlargement
Myocardial weakness
Oak poisoning (ventral)
Ostertagiasis type 2 (submandibular)
Oxalate poisoning (chronic – ascites)
Parasitic gastroenteritis (submandibular)
Snakebite (local)
Traumatic pericarditis (later stages)

Oedema can be due to stasis which is seen in chronic venous congestion or where any condition alters the normal circulation of blood to the heart. Hydrostatic oedema occurs when there is excess of blood fluids or the blood vessels become excessively porous. This leads to the accumulation of transudate. Inflammatory oedema can occur and may be local or general.

Table 5.6 Some causes of a jugular pulse

Aortic valve insufficiency (sometimes only a diastolic pulse)
Atrioventricular valve insufficiency, right (systolic pulse)
Atrioventricular valve stenosis, right or left
Congestive heart failure
Endocarditis
Enzootic bovine leukosis (cardiac form)
Haemothorax
Hydrothorax
Pericarditis
Post-parturient haemoglobinuria
Sporadic bovine leukosis (thymic form)
Traumatic pericarditis

6 Respiratory system

Nasal discharge
Cough
Larynx and trachea
Examination of the thorax
  Palpation
  Percussion
  Auscultation
  Thoracocentesis
  Radiography
  Endoscopic examination
Rhinitis
Laryngitis
Tracheitis/bronchitis
Pneumonia
Pulmonary congestion/oedema
Pulmonary emphysema
Respiratory problems in calves
Respiratory problems in growing cattle
Respiratory problems in adult cattle

Nasal discharge

The presence of abnormal nasal discharge usually indicates respiratory disease (Table 6.1). However it does also occur where other systemic states make the animal feel dull and disinclined to undertake routine grooming habits such as clearing its nares. The discharge may be mucoid or purulent and usually indicates infection of the nasal cavities or nasal sinuses. A unilateral nasal discharge suggests a local disease process whereas one involving both nasal passages suggests a more generalized problem.

Nasal cavities and sinuses

The examination involves inspection of the face, nose and lips, mucous membranes and the sinuses. The sinuses are examined by inspection, percussion and if necessary exploratory trephin-

Table 6.1 Some causes of nasal discharge

Anaphylaxis (severe – cream, frothy)
Anthrax (blood)
Blue tongue
Bovine malignant catarrh (mucopurulent haemorrhage)
Bovine viral diarrhoea (mucopurulent)
Bracken poisoning (blood)
Cuffing pneumonia (mucopurulent)
Enzootic pneumonia (mucopurulent)
Fat cow syndrome (beef)
Fog fever
Infectious bovine rhinotracheitis (severe)
Iodism
Mucosal disease (mucopurulent)
Oxalate poisoning (acute – blood-tinged)
Pantothenic acid deficiency
Parasitic bronchitis (acute)
Pasteurellosis (pneumonic – mucopurulent)
Pulmonary congestion (slight to moderate serous)
Pulmonary emphysema (intermittent – fluid mucus, mucopurulent)
Pulmonary oedema (slight to moderate)
Pulmonary oedema – severe (voluminous frothy discharge, blood tinged)
Rhinitis (mucosal or purulent)
Rinderpest (serous then purulent)
Salmonellosis
Selenium/vitamin E deficiency (frothy, blood-stained)
Sodium chloride poisoning (acute)
Summer snuffles (yellow tinge)

ing. Percussion in a normal animal gives a full, resonant sound, it becomes duller if the sinuses are partially or completely blocked by mucus or other material. Pain may also be elicited. The submaxillary lymph nodes should be examined for size and consistency.

Cough (Table 6.2)

Coughing is a reflex action aroused by irritation in the mucous membranes of the trachea and bronchi. The action is to remove

Table 6.2 Some causes of coughing

Abomasal dilatation (rare)
Anaphylaxis (severe)
Aspiration pneumonia
Bovine viral diarrhoea (harsh, dry)
Bronchitis
Bronchopneumonia (moist, painful)
Congestive heart failure (left)
Contagious bovine pleuropneumonia
Cuffing pneumonia (calves – harsh, dry)
Diphtheria – calf (laryngeal form – moist, painful)
Enzootic pneumonia (moist)
Infectious bovine rhinotracheitis (short, explosive)
Interstitial pneumonia (dry hack, often paroxysmal)
Laryngitis
Lungworm infestation (acute)
Lungworm infestation (subacute – paroxysmal)
Milk allergy
Mucosal disease (harsh, dry)
Oesophageal obstruction
Oesophagitis
Pasteurellosis (pneumonic – low productive)
Pharyngeal paralysis (mainly when eating)
Pharyngeal phlegmon
Pharyngitis (may be paroxysmal if activated)
Pleurisy
Pneumonia
Pulmonary abscess (marked, short, harsh, painful)
Pulmonary neoplasia
Pulmonary oedema (soft, moist)
Rinderpest
Thrombosis of vena cava
Tracheitis
Tuberculosis
Mycobacterium bovis (low, moist, suppressed)
Mycobacterium avium
Winter dysentery (harsh, occasionally occurs)

foreign material including exudate from the pharynx, larynx, trachea and bronchi. Coughing in animals is involuntary and indicates the presence of an abnormality. The reflex is dependent on impulses from the tracheobronchial tree via the vagus to the coughing centre of the medulla. The nature of the cough is characterized by its frequency, pain, duration, depth, cough sounds or expectoration. In normal cattle, pinching the upper trachea will not elicit a cough. Thus when it occurs it indicates probable respiratory disease. Frequency depends on the degree of the stimulus and tends to be more common the more exudation and inflammation there is in the air spaces. There can be paroxysmal coughing, a continuous cough or fits of coughing. When a cough is painful the animal attempts to suppress it and will often show distress when coughing. This is seen in acute inflammation. The force of the cough can be strong if it is subacute. It tends to be weak if there is a painful condition present or decreased elasticity of the lungs. The duration of the cough normally depends on the force and tends to be a lot longer in a weak cough. The depth of the cough depends on how much air is expelled and can be either shallow or deep. The sounds produced will depend on the force with which the air is expired and can be soft, loud, moist, dry, clear, dull or low. If material is brought up it is at once swallowed.

Larynx and trachea

These are examined by inspection, palpation and auscultation. It is possible to examine the larynx and trachea by endoscope and such inspection can be rewarding. Palpation will indicate any abnormal swellings. Usually auscultation of the larynx reveals stenotic sounds rather like those in the bronchi on inspiration and expiration. In the trachea there is a blowing sound as air passes in and out.

Examination of the thorax

This examination includes palpation, percussion, auscultation, thoracocentesis and radiography.

Palpation

This is of limited value but does allow determination of the nature of any swelling. It can provide indirect evidence such as pain or sensitivity of the thoracic wall and the intercostal spaces. It is most often encountered in problems like pleurisy.

Percussion

The percussion area is deceptively small and the diaphragm is convex (see Figure 6.1). The area is triangular in shape and is severely reduced because of the heavy back musculature, the shoulder muscles and caudally by the abdominal organs. The upper line extends backwards from the caudal angle of the scapula; the cranial limit is from the olecranon process of the ulna to the posterior angle of the sternum; and the third line extends from the olecranon process to the penultimate intercostal space.

When percussion is undertaken in the normal way there is good resonance. However, the success of this exercise depends on the nature of the animal, so that if cattle are fat it is of limited use. The area of percussion can be divided into three, the upper, middle and lower thirds. On the left, in the upper third, the resonance of the lung merges with the upper part of the rumen where fluid is usually present. In the middle third the resonance ceases abruptly due to the solid mass of feed in the rumen. The lower cranial two-thirds is occupied by cardiac dullness and the remaining part contains so little lung tissue that resonance is not heard. On the right side the resonance of the upper third ends

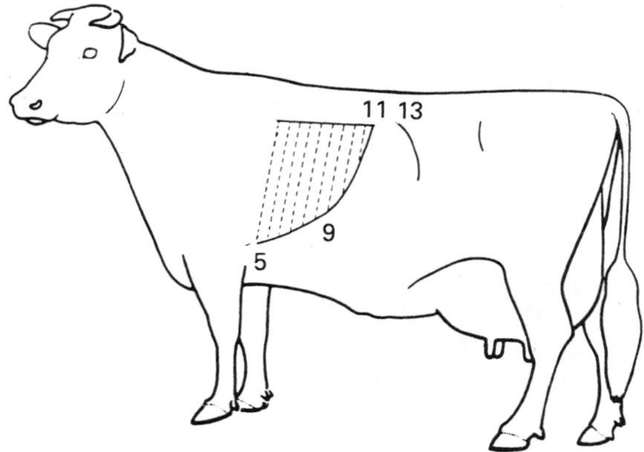

Figure 6.1 Area of percussion of thorax in cow: 5, fifth rib; 9, ninth rib; 11, eleventh intercostal space; 13, thirteenth rib. From *Clinical Diagnosis of Diseases of Large Animals*, W.J. Gibbons (1966). Philadelphia, Lea & Febiger

abruptly due to the liver. In the middle third the resonance is pronounced cranially but reduces more rapidly than the upper third when percussion continues caudally. In the lower third there is less area of cardiac dullness than on the left and so some resonance from the lung may be elicited. Reduction in resonance may be over the whole thoracic area or just over a specific part. A reduction in resonance occurs with acute congestion of the lungs and consolidation also causes a marked reduction. An increased resonance may suggest emphysema. If percussion reveals tympany, this may be due to pneumothorax or a diaphragmatic hernia with penetration of gas-filled viscera.

Auscultation

Undertaken with the stethoscope, essentially the area of auscultation is similar to that of percussion.

Normal vesicular respiratory sound is heard in both inspiration and expiration. It is a soft murmur and is slightly louder on inspiration than expiration. Vesicular sounds are heard over most of the lung area but are modified over the cardiac area. The sounds tend to be softer in beef cattle and the expiratory sound is almost imperceptible in most cattle.

Bronchial sounds are heard over the lung and trachea. They are blowing in nature and start and finish abruptly. The inspiratory and expiratory sounds are separated by a short pause but are both of roughly the same duration. The normal bronchial sounds are mainly heard where there are large bronchi relatively close to the chest wall. This is normally in the cranial part of the middle third of the auscultation area.

Vesicular sounds can alter in character and can become exaggerated and harsh in nature. These increased sounds may simply be due to exercise or hot conditions. They are also heard when there is a fever or they are reflexly stimulated by pain (Table 6.3). In pneumonia there is increased respiratory effort but this does not create any adventitious sounds. Vesicular sounds are also exaggerated when the healthy area of the lung tries to compensate for abnormal areas, as in pleuritic effusion, pneumonic consolidation, tuberculosis or neoplasia. Harsh vesicular sounds are also heard in interstitial emphysema and bronchitis.

The sounds may be interrupted and jerky if the animal has a fever and these sounds occur over the whole auscultatory area on both sides. A decrease in vesicular sounds occurs where air does not enter the alveoli. In pleurisy with much fluid the

Table 6.3 Some causes of vesicular murmur

Anaphylaxis
Bronchopneumonia
Interstitial pneumonia
Parasitic bronchitis
Pasteurellosis (pneumonic)
Pleurisy
Pneumonia
Pneumothorax (complete collapse)
Pulmonary congestion
Pyrexia

sounds will be almost inaudible. Above the left third level the vesicular sounds are easily heard and may be increased in volume. When there is extensive consolidation then areas with complete absence of sounds will be found (Table 6.4).

Bronchial sounds (Table 6.5) tend to extend into other parts of the lung where there are conditions resulting in less air in the lungs than normal. This means incubation of sound by the lung tissue is enhanced and thus extension of bronchial sounds

Table 6.4 Lung sounds – some causes of dullness

Aspiration pneumonia
Contagious bovine pleuropneumonia
Fog fever
Lungworm infestation (calves)
Pulmonary abscess
Pulmonary neoplasia
Thrombosis of vena cava
Tuberculosis (*Mycobacterium bovis*)

Table 6.5 Some causes of bronchial lung sounds

Atypical interstitial pneumonia
Cuffing pneumonia (calves)
Enzootic pneumonia (calves)
Fog fever
Parasitic bronchitis
Pasteurellosis (pneumonic)
Pneumonia (if consolidation)
Pulmonary congestion
Pulmonary oedema

occurs in lung consolidation. If consolidation of the area is complete then only bronchial sounds will occur. However, if only part of the area is involved then the bronchial sounds are superimposed on the vesicular sounds. Vague tones or sounds are sometimes heard and are called bronchovesicular breathing. These occur in the early or incomplete stages of lung consolidation.

Adventitious sounds or râles are abnormal sounds arising from disease of the bronchi, lungs or pleura. They are in four categories: dry sounds, moist sounds, crepitations and friction sounds.

Dry râles (Table 6.6) are the result of air moving over the mucous membranes of abnormal bronchi and by exudate on the mucosa. This sets up a vibration and the sounds vary in pitch according to the size of the tube in which they occur. They are known as musical râles or rhonchi. Through the large bronchi the sounds are low-pitched, like a deep hum or snore and are known as sonorous. In the small bronchi the sounds are higher-pitched or squeaky whistling and are called sibilant.

Moist sounds (Table 6.7) can be produced in the bronchi, bronchioles or alveoli. These are heard as bubbling sounds and indicate the presence of fluid such as mucus, transudate, pus or blood. Moist râles are relatively consistent and are usually short breathing sounds produced by less copious or viscid fluid. The sounds tend to be removed by coughing or dyspnoea. Moist sounds are well recognized in bronchitis and bronchopneumonia. The signs can be further classified as fine or coarse sounds. Fine breathing râles occur over the fine bronchi and bronchioles. Coarse breathing râles occur over the trachea, bronchial tree and upper bronchi.

Crepitation râles are small multiple crackling sounds produced by passage of air into the alveoli. They are only heard on

Table 6.6 Lung sounds – dry râles (rhonchi)

Atypical interstitial pneumonia
Bronchitis
Cuffing pneumonia (calves)
Enzootic pneumonia (calves)
Laryngitis
Pasteurellosis (pneumonic – later stages)
Pulmonary emphysema
Tracheitis
Tuberculosis (*Mycobacterium bovis*)

Table 6.7 Lung sounds – fluid râles

Anaphylaxis (some cases)
Aspiration pneumonia
Congestive heart failure
Contagious bovine pleuropneumonia
Enzootic pneumonia (calves)
Parasitic bronchitis
Pasteurellosis (pneumonic – early stages)
Pleurisy
Pulmonary oedema
Thrombosis of the vena cava

inspiration and usually towards its end. They are produced by air passing into alveoli which are collapsed or full of fluid. The râles are due to the sudden separation of alveolar walls which have become adherent, usually due to excitation. The walls are drawn apart when sufficient negative pressure has built up. Crepitation is one of the cardinal signs of the first stage of pneumonia but disappears as the lung undergoes consolidation. Crepitation will occur around an area of consolidation if it is surrounded by a zone in which pneumonia is still progressing. It is also heard when the lung is showing resolution and in haemoptysis, pulmonary oedema, aspiration pneumonia and the earlier stages of tuberculosis.

Emphysema (Table 6.8) produces a harsh crackling sound like screwing up a newspaper. The sound is heard throughout inspiration and to a lesser extent during expiration.

When the pleura (Table 6.9) are involved in disease the lung sounds may be dull or toneless. They may have a creaking, rubbing or friction sound when the pleural surfaces are roughened by inflammatory processes but there is not sufficient fluid to separate the visceral and parietal layers. The sounds occur with the respiratory movements but may not be continuous and are not removed by dyspnoea or coughing. They may be loud or widespread depending on the extent of the

Table 6.8 Some causes of emphysema

Anaphylaxis
Fog fever
Lungworm infestation
Pulmonary congestion
Pulmonary emphysema

Table 6.9 Some causes of pleuritic rub

Aspiration pneumonia
Contagious bovine pleuropneumonia
Pasteurellosis (pneumonic)
Pleurisy
Pulmonary emphysema

pleurisy. When a pleurisy is painful the respiratory character is altered and becomes principally abdominal, often with a pleuritic line present. Very occasionally tinkling or metallic sounds occur due to air entering the pleura in pneumothorax or damage to bronchi allowing air to enter the pleural cavity.

Thoracocentesis

Paracentesis of the thoracic cavity is justified if fluid is considered to be present. A needle of about 12.5 cm (5 in) in length and of 10 or 12 gauge is suitable. It should be introduced at the sixth or seventh intercostal space at a level below the anticipated fluid line. The pericardial sac must be avoided. The fluid may contain pus and blood, and direct smears can be examined under the microscope.

Tracheal washes can be of use in cytological and bacteriological examination. A large gauge (10) needle is introduced between two intratracheal rings. A long (60 cm; 15 in) polythene catheter is used and 30 ml sterile saline introduced. It is then collected back. In normal lungs there are citrated epithelia, macronucleocytes and a few neutrophils. When infection is present polymorphs predominate. Occasionally eosinophil numbers are large and this may be due to an allergic or parasitic cause.

Radiography

Radiographic examination is practicable in the very young bullock but it is less feasible in the older animal unless powerful facilities and adequate restraint are available. Contrast media can be helpful in examining the trachea and its patency.

Endoscopic examination

A fibreoptic endoscope can be used to examine the nasal cavity, pharynx, larynx, trachea and major bronchi.

Rhinitis

Although inflammation of the nasal mucous membranes often occurs it is usually part of other disease complexes (Table 6.10).

Table 6.10 Some causes of rhinitis

Viral
Bovine malignant catarrh
Infectious bovine rhinotracheitis
Mucosal disease
Rinderpest
Allergic
Summer snuffles

Laryngitis

This again usually occurs with rhinitis or tracheitis and often with pharyngitis or bronchitis (Table 6.11).

Table 6.11 Some causes of laryngitis

Viral
Infectious bovine rhinotracheitis
Bacterial
Calf diphtheria (*Fusiformis necrophorus*)
Haemophilus somnus
Other
Laryngeal paralysis

Tracheitis/bronchitis

Both occur commonly but with other disease entities, e.g. infectious bovine rhinotracheitis.

Pneumonia (Table 6.12)

This involves inflammation of the parenchyma of the lungs plus also the bronchioles. Often pleurisy is also present.

Pulmonary congestion/oedema

This is an accumulation of blood in the lungs due to engorgement of the vascular bed (Table 6.13). It can then be followed by oedema. Cases are unusual.

Table 6.12 Some causes of pneumonia

Bacterial
- *Actinomyces bovis*
- *Actinomyces (Corynebacterium) pyogenes*
- *Chlamydia* spp.
- *Dermatophilus* spp.
- *Escherichia coli*
- *Fusiformis necrophorus*
- *Haemophilus somnus*
- *Klebsiella pneumoniae*
- *Mycobacterium bovis*
- *Mycobacterium tuberculosis*
- *Pasteurella haemolytica*
- *Pasteurella multocida*
- *Pseudomonas* spp.
- *Streptococcus* spp.

Mycoplasmal
- *Acholeplasma laidlawii*
- *Mycoplasma bovis*
- *Mycoplasma dispar*
- *Mycoplasma mycoides*
- *Ureaplasma*

Mycotic

Parasitic
- *Dictyocaulus viviparus*

Viral
- Adenovirus III
- Bovine viral diarrhoea
- Infectious bovine rhinotracheitis
- Parainfluenza III
- Reovirus I
- Respiratory syncytial virus
- Rhinovirus

Table 6.13 Some causes of pulmonary congestion and/or oedema

Physical
- Irritation by smoke, gas fumes

Other disease problems
- Anaphylaxis
- Congestive heart failure
- Fog fever
- Hypostatic congestion (recumbency)
- Mastitis (coliform)
- Organophosphorus poisoning
- Pneumonia (early stages)

Pulmonary emphysema (Table 6.14)

This is overdistension of the lung due to obstruction of the alveoli with air. This leads to alveolar rupture and air may enter the interstitial spaces. It is a condition secondary to other problems.

Table 6.14 Some causes of pulmonary emphysema

Disease problems
Anaphylaxis
Atypical interstitial pneumonia
Atelectasis (calves)
Chlorine gas poisoning
Fog fever
Parasitic bronchitis
Pneumonia
Pulmonary abscess
Pulmonary oedema
Toxaemia (severe)
Traumatic reticulitis
Welding fumes

Table 6.15 Differential diagnosis of some respiratory problems in calves

Condition	*Signs*
Neonatal acute respiratory distress syndrome	Some dyspnoea
Congenital heart problems	Often small calf, usually systolic murmur, cyanosis
Pulmonary abscess following septicaemia	Often swollen navel, pyrexia, non-respiratory signs
Acidosis following enteritis	Enteritis for a day or so, dehydration, tachycardia
Inhalation pneumonia	Toxaemia, moist râles, often areas of dullness
Acute exudative pneumonia	Pyrexia, some moist sounds, pleuritic rub
Chronic (cuffing) pneumonia	Bright, eating, single dry cough, dry lung sounds
Acute (enzootic) pneumonia	Pyrexia, some dullness, moist and dry sounds
Infectious bovine rhinotracheitis (respiratory)	Pyrexia, conjunctivitis, explosive cough, nasal lesions
Calf diphtheria (laryngeal)	Stertor, dyspnoea, painful cough, painful laryngeal area
Chronic suppurative bronchial pneumonia	Dull, poor weight gain, recurrent respiratory sounds. Moist sounds and areas of dullness
Dusty feed rhinotracheitis	Coughing following feeding, oculonasal discharge, bright
Tuberculosis	Often no signs, but may be soft moist cough, stertor, loss of condition

From *Calf Management and Disease Notes*, A. H. Andrews (1983), published by the Author, Welwyn.

Table 6.16 Differential diagnosis of some respiratory problems in growing cattle

Condition	*Signs*
Acidosis	Temperature low or normal, ruminal stasis, tachycardia, yellow diarrhoea
Acute exudative pneumonia	Pyrexia, some moist sounds, pleuritic rub
Anaphylaxis	Dyspnoea, muscle tremors, urticaria, diarrhoea
Aspiration pneumonia	Toxaemia, moist râles, often areas of dullness
Avian tuberculosis	Cough
Bacillary haemoglobinuria	Dyspnoea, terminally diarrhoea
Bovine nasal granuloma	Dyspnoea, stertor, mucopurulent oculonasal discharge, sneezing
Chronic suppurative pneumonia	Loss of condition, thoracic pain, intermittent pyrexia
Dusty feed rhinotracheitis	Coughing following feeding, oculonasal discharge, bright
Ethylenediamine hydroiodide poisoning	Lachrymation, some coughing, pyrexia, nasal discharge
Fluorosis	Dyspnoea, diarrhoea, constipation, muscle tremors, weakness
Fog fever	Dyspnoea, no coughing, dullness
Haemophilus somnus infection	Tachypnoea, hyperpnoea, conjunctivitis
Infectious bovine rhinotracheitis	Pyrexia, conjunctivitis, explosive cough, nasal lesions
Inhalation pneumonia	Toxaemia, moist râles, often areas of dullness
Laryngeal diphtheria	Stertor, dyspnoea, painful cough, painful laryngeal region
Linseed poisoning	Dyspnoea, staggering, dullness, muscle tremors
Malignant catarrhal fever	Dyspnoea, stertor, nervous signs, lymph node enlargement
Monensin poisoning	Dyspnoea, diarrhoea, dullness
Mucosal disease	Mucopurulent discharge from nostrils, diarrhoea
Organophosphorus poisoning	Dyspnoea, salivation, diarrhoea, lachrymation, miosis, bradycardia
Parasitic bronchitis	Loss of condition, dyspnoea, paroxysmal coughing
Shipping fever	Dullness, pyrexia, tachypnoea
Summer snuffles	Dyspnoea, stertor, mucopurulent oculonasal discharge, sneezing

Table 6.16 continued

Condition	Signs
Thrombosis of caudal/cranial vena cava	Haemoptysis, tachypnoea, melaena, thoracic pain
Tuberculosis (bovine)	Soft chronic cough, tachypnoea, hyperpnoea, dyspnoea
Urea poisoning	Dyspnoea, bloat, abdominal pain
Vitamin E/selenium deficiency	Hyperpnoea, dyspnoea, myoglobinuria
Yew poisoning	Dyspnoea, muscle tremors, weakness, collapse

From *Growing Cattle Management and Disease Notes – Part 2 Disease*, A. H. Andrews (1986), published by the Author, Welwyn.

Table 6.17 Differential diagnosis of some respiratory problems in adult cattle

Condition	Signs
Acidosis	Temperature low or normal, ruminal stasis, tachycardia, yellow diarrhoea
Acute exudative pneumonia	Pyrexia, some moist sounds, pleuritic rub
Anaphylaxis	Dyspnoea, muscle tremors, urticaria, diarrhoea
Aspiration pneumonia	Toxaemia, moist râles, often areas of dullness
Avian tuberculosis	Cough
Bacillary haemoglobinuria	Dyspnoea, terminally diarrhoea
Bovine farmer's lung (insidious)	Severe hyperpnoea, dyspnoea with some mouth breathing, alert
Bovine farmer's lung (sudden onset)	Hyperpnoea, tachypnoea, frequent coughing, decreased milk yield
Bovine nasal granuloma	Dyspnoea, stertor, mucopurulent oculonasal discharge, sneezing
Chronic suppurative pneumonia	Loss of condition, thoracic pain, intermittent pyrexia
Diffuse fibrosing alveolitis	Hyperpnoea, frequent cough, bright, thin, dyspnoea on exercise
Dusty feed rhinotracheitis	Coughing following feeding, oculonasal discharge, bright
Ethylenediamine hydroiodide poisoning	Lachrymation, some coughing, pyrexia, nasal discharge

Table 6.17 continued

Condition	*Signs*
Fluorosis	Dyspnoea, diarrhoea, constipation, muscle tremors, weakness
Fog fever	Dyspnoea, no coughing, dullness
Haemophilus somnus infection	Tachypnoea, hyperpnoea, conjunctivitis
Infectious bovine rhinotracheitis	Pyrexia, conjunctivitis, explosive cough, nasal lesions
Inhalation pneumonia	Toxaemia, moist râles, often areas of dullness
Linseed poisoning	Dyspnoea, staggering, dullness, muscle tremors
Malignant catarrhal fever	Dyspnoea, stertor, nervous signs, lymph node enlargement
Monensin poisoning	Dyspnoea, diarrhoea, dullness
Mucosal disease	Mucopurulent discharge from nostrils, diarrhoea
Organophosphorus poisoning	Dyspnoea, salivation, diarrhoea, lachrymation, miosis, bradycardia
Parasitic bronchitis	Loss of condition, dyspnoea, paroxysmal coughing
Pasteurellosis	Dullness, pyrexia, tachypnoea
Reinfection husk syndrome	Tachypnoea, some hyperpnoea, coughing
Summer snuffles	Dyspnoea, stertor, mucopurulent oculonasal discharge, sneezing
Thrombosis of caudal/cranial vena cava	Haemoptysis, tachypnoea, melaena, thoracic pain
Tuberculosis (bovine)	Soft chronic cough, tachypnoea, hyperpnoea, dyspnoea
Urea poisoning	Dyspnoea, bloat, abdominal pain
Yew poisoning	Dyspnoea, muscle tremors, weakness, collapse

From: *Adult Cattle Management and Disease Notes*, A. H. Andrews (not yet published).

7 Urinary system

Rectal examination
Catheterization
Urinalysis
Renal function tests
Blood samples
Nephrosis

The urinary system is uncommonly affected in cattle disease. Urination is reflex and is dependent on the activation of receptors in the bladder with stretching and contraction of the musculature. Examination of micturition can be helpful in that changes in posture suggest possible painful areas or interference with muscular control. Causes of polyuria are shown in Table 7.1. There may be pain or more frequent micturition (Table 7.2). The frequency of micturition is dependent on the fluid intake (Table 7.3).

Anuria is a cessation of urine flow, as occurs with the presence of urethral calculi. Polyuria is where micturition is more frequent and it is unusual in cattle unless they are receiving diuretics. Stranguria is where there are frequent attempts to urinate with only a small volume of urine being passed; vaginitis is a cause of such a problem. Painful urination or dysuria is indicated by restlessness. Often attempts are made to reduce or stop urine flow so that it comes out in an interrupted stream or as small drops of urine; this occurs in urethritis, vaginitis or cystitis. Ischuria is abnormal retention of urine due to increased distension of the bladder and incidence is uncommon in cattle. However, it can occur with urethral calculi.

Table 7.1 Some causes of polyuria

Contagious pyelonephritis
Ergot poisoning (chronic)
Nephrosis (chronic)
Oak poisoning
Ochratoxin A poisoning
Sodium deficiency
Sodium chloride poisoning

Table 7.2 Some causes of frequent micturition

Chlorinated hydrocarbon poisoning
Contagious bovine pleuronephritis
Cystitis
Oleander poisoning
Oxalate poisoning (acute)
Urethritis
Urolithiasis

Table 7.3 Some causes of polydipsia

Abomasal ulceration with perforation
Abomasitis (acute)
Acetonaemia (some cases)
Amyloidosis
Cereal engorgement (unusual sign)
Circulation failure, peripheral
Contagious pyelonephritis
Copper poisoning (chronic)
Displaced abomasum (right-sided)
Ergot poisoning (calves)
Fever
Hepatitis
Johne's disease
Ochratoxin A poisoning
Phosphorus poisoning
Salmonellosis (acute enteritis)
Sodium deficiency
Septicaemia

Rectal examination

This is the best method of determining kidney or bladder abnormalities. Palpation of the urethra is of only limited value.

Catheterization

It is possible to catheterize the urethra of a cow with a fairly rigid catheter of about 0.5 cm diameter. A finger is inserted into the suburethral diverticulum and the catheter passed over the top of it into the external urethral orifice. While it is possible to pass a catheter in a bull or steer, it is difficult and damage and infection can occur because of difficulties in traversing the sigmoid flexure.

Urinalysis

It is not always easy to collect urine but a nervous animal will often urinate during a clinical examination. Catheterization can be helpful in the cow but is virtually impossible in the male. Two people on either side of the animal holding hands and then putting pressure in front of the udder will often result in urine flow.

Quantity

The urine can be examined for quantity but this mainly depends on the assessor's observation powers. Usually between 4.5 and 19 litres are voided daily.

Colour

The colour is usually pale yellow to brown. It becomes darker in colour when it is retained or is reduced in quantity. The colour can be red, brown-red or brown-black if problems have arisen. These include haematuria (Table 7.4), haemoglobinuria (Table 7.5) and myoglobinuria (Table 7.6). Haematuria will settle out on standing whereas in haemoglobinuria the colour remains red.

Transparency

The urine of cattle is transparent when passed. It may become cloudy if it is allowed to stand. It is also cloudy if pus, bacteria, fat, blood or spermatozoa are present.

Odour

The odour of cattle urine is not unpleasant when fresh. However, if it is retained it becomes more fetid. It also tends to smell if there is cystitis due to bacteria producing ammonia. A smell of acetones may be apparent in ketosis.

Table 7.4 Some causes of haematuria

Pre-renal
- Bracken poisoning
- Kidney trauma
- Purpura haemorrhagica
- Septicaemia

Renal
- Embolism of the renal artery/renal infarction
- Embolic nephritis
- Glomerulonephritis (acute)
- Pyelonephritis
- Tubular damage due to sulphonamide treatment

Post-renal
- Acute cystitis
- Enzootic haematuria
- Urolithiasis

Table 7.5 Some causes of haemoglobinuria

Babesiasis
Bacillary haemoglobinuria
Blood transfusion reaction
Bracken poisoning
Chronic copper poisoning
Cold water intoxication (calves)
Enterotoxaemia (calves)
Eperythrozoonoisis (mainly Africa)
Internal haemorrhage
Isoimmunization haemolytic anaemia of newborn
Kale poisoning
Leptospirosis
Mercury poisoning
Onion poisoning
Post-parturient haemoglobinuria
Rape poisoning
Shipping fever (mainly America)
Sweet clover poisoning (America)

Table 7.6 Some causes of myoglobinuria

Muscle damage
Muscular dystrophy
Selenium deficiency
Vitamin E deficiency

Specific gravity

The normal specific gravity is 1.020–1.045. However, a high specific gravity occurs when the animal reduces its fluid production.

pH

Usually cattle excrete alkaline urine due to the presence of soluble calcium bicarbonate. In febrile conditions and where there is anorexia the urine will become acid. Abnormally alkaline urine with ammonia production from urea occurs in cystitis.

Protein

Protein in high levels occurs where the glomerular matrix allows proteins to enter the filtrate. It occurs in nephritis and congestive heart failure as well as in cattle which have been recumbent.

Deposits

If urine is spun down there may be cellular debris, calculi, spermatozoa, leucocytes, erythrocytes. Casts can be produced as cylindrical moulds of the renal tubules.

Bile pigments

The overproduction of bile pigments can lead to the induction of hepatic cell damage as well as bile duct stasis.

Glucose

Glucose in the urine is uncommon in cattle but does occur in diabetes mellitus.

Ketones

Some ketone bodies can be present in the urine of normal cattle. Large quantities do however occur in ketosis.

Renal function tests

The most effective way of measuring the ability of the kidneys to function is to determine whether it is possible for the animal to alter the specific gravity of its urine. Thus the specific gravity ought to increase if the animal is deprived of water.

Blood samples

These are only of much value when there has been considerable damage to the kidney nephrons. In such cases, blood urea, non-protein nitrogen and creatinine content will all rise. However it should be realized that urea does rise if there is much protein being digested or catabolism is occurring.

Nephrosis

This indicates conditions which result in a degeneration or inflammation of the renal tubules. Conditions involved can be acute or chronic (Table 7.7).

Table 7.7 Some causes of nephrosis

Toxins
Calcium salt overdosage
Chlorinated naphthalene poisoning
Mercury poisoning
Sulphonamide poisoning
Toxaemia

8 Nervous system

Techniques of examination
History
Examination
Cranial nerves
Peripheral nerves
Spinal reflexes
Spinal examination
Ophthalmoscopic examination
Cerebrospinal fluid examination
Putative genetic neurological disorders in calves
Putative genetic neurological disorders in growing cattle
Putative genetic neurological disorders in adult cattle
Central nervous problems in calves
Central nervous problems in growing cattle
Central nervous problems in adult cattle

While the nervous system can be the primary source of disease problems, it can also be secondarily affected, particularly where nutritional disturbances interfere with its function. Diagnosis of neurological conditions always produces an intellectual and diagnostic challenge and it would be fair to say that methods of large animal neurology have not been developed to anything like the same extent as those in human or small animal medicine. This is obviously mainly because of economics, although much of the fundamental work on basic neurology is not as advanced as with small animals.

In all cases, because of the lack of examination techniques, a good history is required. Where the disease is limited to a single animal the main problem is to distinguish whether or not it is likely to be the first of many or just an individual condition. Nervous disease can be divided into functional and structural. Those of the functional group are where no lesion can be demonstrated macroscopically or histologically.

The normal purpose of the nervous system is to maintain the body in its environment. The system reacts to stimuli internally and externally. It has several different parts involving the autonomic nervous system which controls the activity of smooth muscle and the endocrine organs, the sensoanimation system, which affects among other tissues the striated muscles and is concerned with locomotion and posture, the mainly sensory system of special sensors and finally the psychic system which controls the animal's mental state.

Certain clinical signs can indicate that the nervous system is affected. These include:

1. *Disturbances of consciousness*. There may be either a decrease or increase in mental awareness. The disturbances often include the cerebrum and include depression states such as dullness, somnolence, lassitude, syncope and coma.
2. *Involuntary muscle movements*. These occur if there are disturbances in the motor centre of the brain. They can result in varying degrees of intensity. Thus there may be fine twitching muscle tremors, convulsions (including clonic spasms, tonic spasms, tetanic spasms) and enforced movement. If the muscle areas are very small it may result in skin twitching and hence movements are fibrillating. In other cases muscle groups may be affected and may actually result in movements of the limbs, head, etc. When these occur they may be increased when the animal does move or tense for any reason and this is often an indication of cerebellar involvement.

3. *Disturbances of posture and mobility.* When disturbances of posture occur due to nervous disease they are rarely continuous. They can include head pressing, opisthotonus, deviation of head or neck, rotation of the head, etc. Many of the abnormalities of mobility include paresis and paralysis. Paresis results in the animal being unable to rise whereas paralysis indicates a more local condition and can be due to local nerve damage. Ataxia or incoordination of the gait is often the result of cerebellar dysfunction and it can be difficult to differentiate from partial paralysis and proprioceptive dysfunction.
4. *Disturbances of sensation.* Lesions diagnosed in animals may involve sight and the vestibular apparatus. Where there are lesions of the peripheral sensory neurons there is hypersensitivity or reduced sensation. Tests to determine sensitivity are difficult to interpret as failure to respond to a painful stimulus can be due to the variation between normal individuals as well as failure to perceive the stimulus or inability to respond.
5. *Disturbances of coordination.* Those involving the brain are uncommon in animals and are often an overlap with disturbances of motility.
6. *Disturbances of the autonomic nervous system.* Affections of the autonomic nervous system are of considerable importance in cattle. Lesions can occur cranially or spinally. Those involving the cranial parasympathetic outflow involve abnormalities in constriction of the pupils, salivating and the involuntary muscular activity of the upper respiratory tract and upper alimentary tract. There is usually involvement of the oculomotor (III), facial (VII), glossopharyngeal (IX) and vagus (X) nerves or their nuclei. When the craniocervical branch of the sympathetic system is involved there is interference with pupillary constriction and salivation. Problems of the spinal sympathetic system involve the natural motility of the heart, alimentary tract and other viscera. Central lesions of the hypothalamus can result in problems of obesity or heat exchange such as hyperthermia of hypothermia.

Techniques of examination

History

Much useful information can be gained from careful history-taking. This involves the breed, age, sex, as well as diet, dietary changes and any recent management changes. Other incidents such as calving, castrating, dehorning, housing or turnout should be included.

Examination

Ideally the animal should at first be examined undisturbed in the environment in which it is being kept. Its relationship with others in its group should be noted. Any changes in behaviour and attitude should also be noted. Some of the signs and their possible importance are shown in Table 8.1.

Movement within the group may give an indication if incoordination or ataxia occur sporadically. If the animal is then

Table 8.1 Alteration in carriage of the head and its likely indication

Signs	*Principal area of lesion*
Head tilt (rotation on the long axis)	Middle ear Inner ear disease Vestibular nuclei of medulla (lesion usually on the same site as lower ear)
Head deviation (lateral, downward or upward)	Cortical lesions (usually) Brain stem lesions
Head tremor (vertical or horizontal) Low frequency	Cerebellar problems Diencephala problems
Head tremor (vertical or horizontal) High frequency	Encephalitis Congenital intracranial malfunction
Circling movements	Brain stem lesion Cerebellar lesion (both on side to which animal turns) Cerebral lesion (usually side opposite to which animal turns)
Head symmetry: facial paralysis	Medullary lesion Facial nerve (VII) damage
Nystagmus	Pons lesions Mid-brain lesion Cerebellum lesion Inner ear problem
Uneven pupillary size	Paralysis of parasympathetic (constrictor) pathway from upper brain stem Paralysis of sympathetic (dilator) pathways

From Barlow, R. M. (1983). *In Practice* 5, May, 77–84.

separated from the others, this provides useful information. It will indicate possible coordination, balance and sight troubles.

The tones of skeletal muscles may alter and there may also be muscular wasting.

Table 8.2 Some causes of blindness

Acetonaemia (apparent)
Aflatoxicosis
Brain abscess
Brain neoplasia
Cerebrocortical necrosis
Clostridium perfringens type D
Coenurosis (unilateral – some cases)
Electrocution
Endocarditis
Ergot poisoning, acute (intermittent)
Gid (unilateral – some cases)
Haemophilus somnus infection (often unilateral)
Infectious bovine rhinotracheitis (uncommon sign)
Kale poisoning
Lead poisoning
Lightning strike
Meningitis (cerebral)
Photosensitization (severe)
Ragwort poisoning (partial)
Selenium poisoning
Sodium chloride poisoning (acute)
Vitamin A deficiency

Table 8.3 Some causes of partial blindness

Acetonaemia
Acidosis
Bovine spongiform encephalopathy (possibly)
Brain abscess (some cases)
Brain neoplasia (some cases)
Brain trauma
Cereal engorgement
Metaldehyde poisoning
Vitamin A deficiency

Table 8.4 Some causes of circling

Acetonaemia (nervous)
Aflatoxicosis
Aujeszky's disease
Brain abscess (some cases)
Cerebrocortical necrosis

Table 8.4 continued

Coenurosis
Encephalitis
Gid
Hepatitis
Hydrocephalus (early stages)
Lead poisoning (subacute)
Listeria infection (meningoencephalitis)
Otitis media
Ragwort poisoning
Selenium poisoning

Table 8.5 Some causes of convulsions

Anthrax
Arsenic poisoning (chronic)
Bovine malignant catarrh
Brain abscess (intermittent)
Brain neoplasia (some cases)
Brain trauma (chronic)
Carbon tetrachloride poisoning (clonic–tonic)
Cerebral anoxia (acute, chronic)
Cerebrocortical necrosis (clonic–tonic)
Circulatory failure, congestive (clonic)
Clostridium perfringens type D
Coccidiosis
Coenurosis (some epileptiform)
Encephalitis (clonic–tonic)
Ergot poisoning, acute (epileptiform)
Familial convulsions (calves)
Fluorosis, acute (tetanic)
Foot-and-mouth disease (cardiac form)
Gid (some epileptiform)
Haemophilus somnus infection
Heart failure (acute clonic)
Hepatitis (some cases)
Hydrocyanic acid poisoning (clonic)
Hypomagnesaemia
Infectious bovine rhinotracheitis (uncommon finding)
Inherited idiopathic epilepsy (epileptiform, calves)
Laburnum poisoning
Lead poisoning (clonic–tonic)
Louping ill
Lupin poisoning (clonic)
Mercury poisoning (acute clonic)
Nitrate/nitrite poisoning (clonic)
Oleander poisoning
Organophosphorus poisoning
Penitrem A poisoning (tetanic)
Phosphorus poisoning
Pyridoxine deficiency (epileptiform – calves)

Table 8.5 continued

Ryegrass staggers (tetanic)
Sodium chloride poisoning (clonic)
Strychnine poisoning (tetanic)
Tetanus (tetanic)
Thiamine deficiency
Vitamin A deficiency (clonic–tonic)
Water hemlock poisoning (tetanic)
Water intoxication (clonic–tonic)

Table 8.6 Some causes of incoordination

Arsenic poisoning
Botulism
Bovine malignant catarrh
Bovine spongiform encephalopathy
Cerebellar anoxia
Cerebellar hypoplasia
Chlorinated hydrocarbon poisoning
Crude oil poisoning
Encephalitis
Hemlock poisoning
Hypomagnesaemia
Infectious bovine rhinotracheitis (calf encephalitis)
Laburnum poisoning
Lead poisoning (subacute)
Louping ill
Mercury poisoning (chronic)
Metaldehyde poisoning
Parturient paresis (early stages)
Rabies
Salmonella septicaemia (*S.dublin*, calves)
Thiamine deficiency
Vitamin A deficiency

Table 8.7 Some causes of muscular rigidity

Cerebrocortical necrosis
Chlorinated hydrocarbon poisoning
Louping ill
Meningitis (neck and head)
Penitrem A poisoning
Streptococcal meningitis (calves)
Tetanus

Table 8.8 Some causes of muscle tremor

Anaphylaxis
Anthrax
Arsenic poisoning
Bovine malignant catarrh
Bovine spongiform encephalopathy
Cerebral anoxia (acute – from head to trunk and limbs)
Cerebral anoxia (chronic)
Cerebrocortical necrosis
Chlorinated hydrocarbon poisoning
Coccidiosis
Encephalitis
Fat cow syndrome
Fluorosis (acute)
Gas gangrene
Haemophilus somnus infection
Hepatitis (some cases)
Hydrocyanic acid poisoning (subacute)
Hypomagnesaemia
Lead poisoning
Louping ill
Malignant oedema
Mannosidosis
Meningitis
Metaldehyde poisoning
Milk allergy
Monochloroacetate poisoning
Nitrate/nitrite poisoning
Oleander poisoning
Organophosphorus poisoning
Oxalate poisoning (acute)
Parturient paresis
Penitrem A toxicity
Selenium/vitamin E deficiency (subacute)
Strychnine poisoning
Sulphur poisoning
Urea poisoning
Water intoxication
Yew poisoning

Table 8.9 Some causes of nystagmus

Anaphylaxis – severe
Bovine malignant catarrh
Brain abscess (some cases)
Brain tumour
Cerebrocortical necrosis
Coccidiosis
Electrocution
Encephalitis

Table 8.9 continued

Haemophilus somnus infection
Hydrocyanic acid poisoning
Hypomagnesaemia
Lightning strike
Listeria infection (septicaemia – calves)
Penitrem A poisoning
Salmonella septicaemia (*S.dublin*, calves)

Table 8.10 Some causes of opisthotonus

Aujeszky's disease
Cerebrocortical necrosis
Clostridium perfringens types A,B,C,D,E
Coccidiosis
Haemophilus somnus infection
Hydrocyanic acid poisoning
Hypomagnesaemia
Lead poisoning
Listeria infection (septicaemia – calves)
Meningitis
Penitrem A poisoning
Strychnine poisoning
Tetanus
Vitamin A deficiency

Table 8.11 Some causes of paralysis

Aujeszky's disease
Biotin deficiency (calves)
Bone fractures, inflammation, etc.
Botulism (flaccid)
Bovine malignant catarrh
Cerebral anoxia (acute – flaccid)
Coenurosis (spinal, gradual)
Electrocution
Enzootic bovine leukosis (nervous form – progressive)
Ergot poisoning (acute – temporary)
Foot-and-mouth disease (unusual form)
Gid (spinal, gradual)
Hydrocephalus (gradual onset, eventually complete)
Lightning strike
Listeriosis
Louping ill
Mercury poisoning
Muscle damage
Nerve damage
Osteodystrophy (due to spinal cord compression)
Oxalate poisoning (acute)

Table 8.11 continued

Photosensitization (severe)
Ryegrass staggers
Selenium poisoning
Sodium chloride poisoning
Spastic syndrome
Spinal cord compression (motor paralysis – progressive, then flaccid or sporadic)
Spinal cord trauma (flaccid)
Sporadic bovine leukosis
Trauma
Vitamin A deficiency
Warble fly infestation

Table 8.12 Some causes of dilated pupils

Cerebral engorgement
Coenurosis (unilateral)
Crude oil poisoning
Fluorosis (acute)
Gid (unilateral)
Hydrocyanic acid poisoning
Lead poisoning
Oleander poisoning
Oxalate poisoning (acute)
Parturient paresis
Vitamin A deficiency

Table 8.13 Some causes of sluggish pupillary reflex

Acidosis
Brain trauma
Cereal engorgement
Cerebrocortical necrosis
Meningitis
Parturient paresis

Cranial nerve examination

The nerves can be divided according to their function into:

I Afferent nerves
Olfactory (I), optic (II), auditory (VIII)
II Efferent nerves
Facial (VII), spinal accessory (XI), hypoglossal (XII)
III Mixed nerves
Oculomotor (III), trochlear (IV), trigeminal (V), abducens (VI), glossopharyngeal (IX), vagus (X).

I Olfactory nerve

The sense of smell is usually impossible to determine in cattle although an animal may not show any appreciation of the presence of food whilst seeing it.

II Optic nerve

Unless the animal is blind the degree of function of sight is hard to judge. The ability of the animal to negotiate objects or enter a box is helpful, particularly in dull or subdued light. Otherwise making the animal close its eyelids and withdrawal of the head as the result of provoking the menace or eye preservation reflex is useful. This is done by poking a finger towards the eye.

III Oculomotor nerve

This is usually examined in conjunction with the trochlear (IV) and abducens (VI) nerves. The oculomotor nerve supplies the main eyeball muscles such as the superior oblique, the lateral rectus and retractor muscles as well as the pupillary constrictor muscle of the lens. Loss of function can be assessed by the pupillary reflex constriction when exposed to bright light. Consensual constriction or contraction of the other eye also occurs but to a lesser extent.

IV Trochlear nerve

This supplies the superior oblique muscle of the eye and when paralysed interferes with downward movement of the eye so that it turns inwards rather than downwards.

V Trigeminal nerve

This consists of three main branches:

1. Ophthalmic which is sensory and supplies sensation to the eye, lachrymal glands, upper eyelid and skin of the temporal region and forehead.
2. Maxillary, also sensory and supplies sensation to the lower eyelid, mucous membrane of the nose, the head and soft palate, the teeth of the upper jaw and the mucous membranes of the nasopharynx.
3. Mandibular, which consists of sensory, motor and secretory fibres and supplies sensation to the lower part of the face,

the side of the face, lower lip, ear, tongue and lower teeth. Motor fibres go to the muscles of mastication, the tensor palati and lesser tympani.

The sensory part can be examined by testing the corneal reflex and sensitivity of the face. The corneal test involves touching the cornea with some soft object resulting in rapid, forceful closing of the eye. A conjunctival test involves lightly touching the eye when it will close. The motor functions principally involve the muscles of mastication and their movements should be examined. Unilateral paralysis results in the muscles of the paralysed side being less prominent than on the healthy side. Loss of secretory function due to fifth nerve paralysis results in a dry mouth.

VI Abductor nerve

This supplies motor fibres to the retractor and lateral rectus muscles of the eyelid. If damaged the eye cannot be moved inwards. The eye may show protrusion and medial deviation.

VII Facial nerve

This is entirely motor in origin but receives some sensory fibres. It provides motor supply to the cheek, lips, face, nostril and external ear. Paralysis results in a typical facile expression when the ear drops on the affected side, the lip is drawn towards the healthy side, the lower lip hangs down on the affected side and saliva dribbles from it. When paralysed the muscles cannot contract in response to noise or stabbing a finger at the eye.

VIII Auditory nerve

This consists of a hearing branch and the vestibular branch which maintains equilibrium. Examining hearing is difficult but can be tested by making a sudden noise out of sight of the animal. Abnormalities of head carriage or balance tend to indicate vestibular involvement. In severe cases there is head rotation.

IX Glossopharyngeal nerve

There are three main branches. The first is sensory and supplies nerves to the mucous membrane of the tympanum and the eustachian tube. The second is motor and goes to the pharyngeal muscles with a sensory part supplying the mucous membrane of the pharynx. The third is sensory to the caudal third of the tongue, the soft palate and the tonsillar region. It is very difficult to test the glossopharyngeal nerve and usually it is only involved in problems which also affect other nerves. Defects of this nerve result in inability to swallow, regurgitation of food through the nostrils and interference with the voice and respiration.

X Vagus

This nerve has a considerable number of connections with other nerves and the sympathetic nervous system. The main branches are:

1. Pharyngeal which supplies the muscles of the pharynx and soft palate. When affected the animal may be unable to swallow and sometimes food is regurgitated through the mouth and nostrils.
2. Anterior laryngeal providing sensory nerves for the floor of the pharynx, oesophageal entrance, cranial part of the larynx and the cricothyroid muscle of the larynx. It also anastomoses with the recurrent laryngeal nerve.
3. Recurrent laryngeal nerve provides fibres to all muscles of the larynx except the cricothyroid. It provides a sensory supply to the trachea and oesophagus and with the anterior laryngeal nerve it provides sensation to the mucous membranes of the larynx. Changes due to this nerve are difficult to detect, although they will alter the position of the vocal cords.
4. Cardiac branches which, when affected, accelerate the heart.
5. Tracheal and oesophageal branches innervate the trachea, oesophagus and large blood vessels. When affected there may be difficulty in swallowing. However the pharyngeal branch of the vagus would also be involved.
6. Bronchial branch supplies the bronchi and blood vessels of the lungs. No signs are usually noted in dysfunction.
7. Dorsal and ventral oesophageal branches pass via the mediastinum and enter the abdomen where they supply most of the abdominal viscera. This results in changes in the digestive system when functioning abnormally.

XI Spinal accessory nerve

This has two parts.

1. Accessory, which supplies motor fibres to the vagus for pharynx and larynx and when abnormal can lead to problems of regurgitation of food and a deep voice.
2. Spinal, which supplies motor fibres to the trapezius and sternocephalic muscle. When paralysed the scapula drops and the head is slightly back towards the unaffected side.

XII Hypoglossal nerve

This is the motor nerve to the tongue. If unilateral paralysis occurs the tongue lies to one side. If bilateral the tongue is limp in the mouth.

Peripheral nerves

These consist of a motor and a sensory component.

Motor activity dysfunction

This is often seen as incoordination of locomotion or alteration in balance. There may be muscular atrophy or a muscular spasm.

Sensory activity dysfunction

The investigation is limited and mainly involves determination of skin sensation to painful stimuli. This can be done by palpation or by the use of a pin or hypodermic needle. There is a quick movement of the cutaneous muscle – the panniculus reflex.

Spinal reflexes

Testing of the motor and sensory function of spinal reflexes is difficult. Some can however be valuable.

Superficial reflexes

Conjunctival reflex, corneal reflex and pupillary reflexes have already been described.

Table 8.14 Useful reflexes for diagnosis of neurological disorders

Reflex	*Elicitation and normal response*	*Failure of normal response may indicate lesions in:*
Fixation	Movement of head and eyes towards a moving object, e.g. falling white handkerchief or tuft of cotton wool	Retina, optic tract rostral brain stem, posterior cerebrum, cranial nerves II, IV, VI or cervical nerves. First attempt usually best in cattle as they are quickly bored
Eye protection	Threatening eye with outstretched finger results in blink. Interpose a transparent sheet between hand and eye to avoid corneal stimulation by air movement	Lesion in retina, optic tract anterior brain stem, posterior cerebrum or VIIth cranial nerve
Photomotor	Closure of eyelids when a bright light is shown into the eye	As above. When light applied obliquely R or L, failure of normal response indicates lesion in contralateral visual cortex
Pupillary	Constriction of pupils when eye exposed to bright light after shading	Lesion in retina, optic tract, brain stem
Nictitating	Touching cornea causes retraction of eyeball and movement of nictitating membrane across eye	Rostral brain stem, cranial nerves III and VI
Oculocardiac	Firm pressure on eyeballs slows heart rate immediately, with immediate recovery when compression discontinued	Brain stem, cranial nerves V and X
Cutaneous	Mild pin prick results in local contraction of panniculus muscle; limb withdrawal. More painful stimulus elicits cerebral response	Local spinal reflex arcs, or if painful stimulus given also in spinothalamic tract
Pedal	Firm pressure on interdigital fold or squeezing of a claw with pincers	As above

From Barlow, R. M. (1983). *In Practice* **5**, May, 77–84.

Perineal reflex. This can be of help in assessing the local spinal reflexes in a recumbent animal. An anal fold is pinched and this will cause a reflex contraction of the perineal musculature if it is intact.

Pedal reflex. This is only of value in recumbent animals. The induction of pain above the toe should lead to withdrawal of the toe.

Deep reflexes

Patellar reflex is usually only of value in younger animals. The stifle should be slightly flexed. The patella ligament is sharply struck with the edge of a firm object or the side of the hand. Contraction of the quadriceps muscle makes the leg jerk forwards.

Tarsal reflex. This can only be tested satisfactorily in the recumbent animal and particularly younger cattle. The hock (tarsus) must be slightly flexed, if difficulty is encountered in doing this then it is probable that the reflex is all right. When flexed the Achilles tendon must be struck sharply. There is then a vigorous contraction of the gastrocnemius muscle.

Organic reflexes

These often cannot be tested but their malfunctions may need to be investigated. These include: circulation, defaecation, deglutition, micturition, respiration, temperature.

Spinal examination

Radiography is only practicable in most cases for calves or younger cattle.

Ophthalmoscopic examination

This can be of use in diagnosis of problems. Thus a retinitis may occur in infection of the cranium and meninges. Papilloedema occurs in some problems causing increased brain pressure.

Cerebrospinal fluid examination

This is only occasionally performed. Lumbar, cisternal and lumbosacral puncture can all be undertaken. Cisternal puncture is easier to perform in young animals.

The cerebrospinal fluid in normal cattle is clear and watery and has a specific gravity of 1.005–1.008, a pH of 7.4–8.0 and a viscosity of 1.019–1.029. Its albumin content is 10–22 g/l and the glucose level is 35–70 mg/100 ml (1.94–3.89 mmol/l). In abnormal cases it tends to be opaque with cellular content. The fluid can be tested for magnesium, phosphorus and chloride. A manometer can be applied to the needle so that CSF pressure can be determined.

Electroencephalography (EEG) could assist in diagnosis of brain disease but is little used. It has been suggested to be suitable for detection of bovine spongiform encephalopathy in live animals.

Table 8.15 Congenital neurological disorders of calves with a putative genetic aetiology

Disease	*Mode*	*(Breeds) and princpal features*
Hydrocephalus	R	(Hol, Her, Ayr, Cha). Premature birth, hydrops amnii. Unable to stand, continuous bawling. Open fontanelles, dilated ventricles (achondroplasia)
Cerebellar hypoplasia	R	(Her, Gue, Hol, Sh, Ayr, Zeb). Inability to stay upright, incoordination, impaired vision, rhythmic head movements. Cerebellum absent or small
Cerebellar hypomyelinogenesis	R	(Sh, Her, Ang). Progressive ataxia, recumbency. White matter of cerebellum a poorly defined, reticulated fibre network; absence of myelin
Neuraxial oedema	R?	(PHer). Inability to stand or raise head. Tetanic spasms induced by external stimuli. Spongy vacuolation of CNS in some cases. Hip dysplasia
Brain oedema	R?	(Her). Coarse muscular contractions, nystagmus. Hydrocephalus and generalized spongy transformation
Microcephaly	?	(Her). Stillborn, small brain, prognathism

Ang, Angus; Ayr, Ayrshire; Bfm, Beefmaster; BrSw, Brown Swiss; Cha, Charolais; Fr, Friesian; Gal, Galloway; Gue, Guernsey; Gr, Murray Grey; Her, Hereford; Hol, Holstein; PHer, Polled Hereford; Sh, Shorthorn; Zeb, Zebu.
R = recessive
D = dominant
From Barlow, R. M. (1983). *In Practice* **5**, May, 77–84.

Table 8.16 Neurological disorders of growing cattle with a putative genetic aetiology

Disease	*Mode*	*(Breeds) and principal features*
Doddler	R	(Her). Incoordination, severe muscular spasms, respiratory difficulty, nystagmus, convulsions. Calcification of cerebellar and medullary neurons
Cerebellar abiotrophy	R?	(Hol). Ataxia, spastic dysmetria, rhythmic head movements. Degeneration of cerebellar neurons
Familial convulsions and ataxia	D	(Ang). Tetanic seizure with ataxia and hypermetria developing later. Rhythmic head movements. Purkinje cell/axon degenerations
Idiopathic epilepsy	D	(Br Sw). Epileptiform seizures triggered by excitement or exercise. Pathology undetermined
Mannosidosis	R	(Ang, Gr, Gal). Progressive ataxia, wasting and aggression, α-mannosidase deficiency. Accumulation of oligosaccharides in neurons, fixed macrophages and some epithelial cells
GM, gangliosidosis	R	(Fr). Reduced growth rate and progressive neuromotor dysfunction. Deficiency of β-galactosidase, glycolipids accumulate in neurons
Generalized Type II glycogenosis	R	(Sh, Her). Muscular weakness; incoordination. Deficiency of α-1.4 glucosidase. Diastase soluble, PAS + granules accumulate in cells of many tissues
Chediak-Higashi	R	(Br Sw). Partial albinism, increased susceptibility to infection. Lipofuscin accumulations in neurons and red blood cells
Neuronal lipodystrophy	R	(Bfm). Blindness and circling. Multilamellar, curvilinear inclusions accumulate in nerve cells and fixed macrophages

Table 8.16 continued

Disease	*Mode*	*(Breeds) and principal features*
Progressive ataxia	R?	(Cha). Hypermetria, muscular weakness incoordination, recumbency, rhythmic head movements. Demyelinated plaques
Periodic spasticity	R	(Hol, Gue). Recurrent spastic attacks lasting up to 30 min. CNS pathology undetermined
Spastic paresis	R?	(Many breeds). Excessive tone of gastrocnemius and perforatus muscles with variable age of onset. Pathology uncertain

Ang, Angus; Ayr, Ayrshire; Bfm, Beefmaster; Br Sw, Brown Swiss; Cha, Charolais; Fr, Friesian; Gal, Galloway; Gue, Guernsey; Gr, Murray Grey; Her, Hereford; Hol, Holstein; PHer, Polled Hereford; Sh, Shorthorn; Zeb, Zebu.
R = recessive
D = dominant
From Barlow, R. M. (1983). *In Practice* 5, May, 77–84.

Table 6.17 Differential diagnosis of central nervous problems in calves

Disease	*Blindness*	*Dullness*	*Hyperaesthesia*	*Pyrexia*	*Other signs*	*Other nervous signs*	*Response to therapy*	*Diagnosis*
Colisepticaemia	No	Yes	Usually no	Yes	Sometimes diarrhoea	Nystagmus, muscle tremors	Occasionally, if early	Zinc sulphate turbidity, blood culture
Salmonella – peracute septicaemia	No	Yes	Usually no	Yes	Sometimes diarrhoea	Nystagmus, incoordination	Occasionally, if early	Faecal swab
Enterotoxaemia	No	Yes	Sometimes	No	Diarrhoea/dysentery	Opisthotonus, tetanus	Very poor	Faecal swab
(*Clostridium perfringens* (*welchii*) types B and C)	No	Yes	Some	Yes	Good condition, diarrhoea	Opisthotonus, tetanus	Poor	Faecal swab toxin presence
Coccidiosis	No	Slight	Yes	No or sight	Diarrhoea/dysentery	Strabismus, tetany, opisthotonus	Poor	Faecal sample
Arsenic poisoning	No	Very	Usually no	No	Abdominal pain, fetid diarrhoea	Incoordination, muscle tremors	Variable	Urine sample
Sodium chloride poisoning	Sometimes	Slight	No	No	Excessive thirst, diarrhoea, abdominal pain	Paresis, fetlock knuckling	Usually good if early	Serum sodium levels
Mercury poisoning	Yes	Yes	No	No	Abdominal pain, diarrhoea	Terminal incoordination, convulsions, recumbency	Variable	Post-mortem kidney mercury levels, history, faeces and urine
Nitrate poisoning	No	Yes	No	No	Dyspnoea, diarrhoea, cyanosis	Muscle tremors, staggering gait	Some success if early	Methaemoglobin

Table 8.17 continued

Disease	*Blindness*	*Dullness*	*Hyperaesthesia*	*Pyrexia*	*Other signs*	*Other nervous signs*	*Response to therapy*	*Diagnosis*
Lead poisoning	Yes	No	Yes	No or slight	Ruminal stasis, diarrhoea	Bellowing, tonic–clonic convulsions, lack of palpebral reflex	Some success	Blood lead levels, liver and kidney post mortem
Selenium poisoning	Yes	Yes chronic	Yes acute	No	Colic, depraved appetite, chronic loss of condition	Head pressing, paralysis	Limited success	Blood and urine levels
Acute furazolidone poisoning	No	No	Yes	No	Few other signs	Convulsions	Limited value	History of usage
Aflatoxicosis	Yes	Yes	No	No	Teeth grinding, jaundice, diarrhoea, tenesmus	Walk in circles	Limited value	Use of groundnut or other feed
Greedy calf	Temporary	No	No	No	Death	Convulsions	Prevention stops	Bucket fed
Infectious bovine rhinotracheitis (nervous)	No	Intermittent	Intermittent	Yes	Anorexia	Incoordination	No therapy	Viral isolation
Tuberculosis meningitis	No	Yes	No	No	Often enlarged lymph nodes	Convulsions	No therapy	Tuberculin test
Urolithiasis	No	Yes	No	No	Straining		Good if early	Signs
Hydrocephalus	Usually	Yes	Usually no	No	Often skeletal deformities		None	Signs
Cerebellar hypoplasia	Yes	Usually	No	No	Few other signs	Recumbent, or if stands, exaggerated movements	None	Seen at birth

Inherited cerebellar ataxia	No	Yes	No	No	Few other signs	Progressive incoordination	None	Seen after birth
Familial ataxia and convulsions	No	No	Yes	No	Few other signs	Stiff gait, opisthotonus, recumbency	None	History, postmortem histology
Spastic paresis	No	No	No	No	Over-straight hock	Abnormal gait	Surgical good	Signs
Mannosidosis	No	Slight	Yes	No	Loss of condition	Fine lateral head tremor, vertical head nodding	None	Low tissue α-mannosidase
Linseed poisoning	No	Yes acute	Yes	No	Cyanosis, dyspnoea	Opisthotonus, nystagmus	Variable	Linseed feeding
Ergot poisoning	At times	At times	At times	No	Diarrhoea	Drowsiness, convulsions	No therapy	Presence of sclerotia in feed
Meningitis	No	At times	At times	Yes	Anorexia	Opisthotonus, spasm of neck muscles, paddling movements	Good if early	Cerebrospinal fluid cell count
Hypomagnesaemic tetany	No	No	Yes	Yes	Increased loud heart rate	Opisthotonus, paddling movements	Good if early	Low blood magnesium levels
Vitamin A deficiency	Yes	No	No	No	Diarrhoea, bran skin scales	Convulsions, syncope	No use if congenital, good if postnatal	Low plasma and liver levels
Clostridium perfringens (welchii) type D	Appear to be	Yes subacute	Yes in acute	Yes	Diarrhoea	Convulsions, bellowing	Very poor	Faecal swab, toxin presence
Cerebrocortical necrosis	Yes	Less severe cases	Yes	No	Normal ruminal movements	Muscle tremors, opisthotonus, pupils respond to light, recumbency	Good if early	Age (usually over 6 months), signs, histology, brain fluorescence

From: *Calf Management and Disease Notes*, A. H. Andrews (1983), published by the Author, Welwyn.

Table 8.18 Differential diagnosis of central nervous problems in growing cattle

Disease	*Blindness*	*Dullness*	*Hyperaesthesia*	*Pyrexia*	*Other signs*	*Other nervous signs*	*Response to therapy*	*Diagnosis*
Acidosis	Apparent	Yes	Yes	No	Ruminal stasis, tachycardia	Head deviation, circling, staggering gait, muscle tremors	Variable	Signs, history
Aflatoxicosis	Yes	Yes	No	No	Teeth grinding, jaundice, diarrhoea, tenesmus	Walk in circles	Limited value	Use of groundnut or other feed
Arsenic poisoning	No	Very	Usually no	No	Abdominal pain, fetid diarrhoea	Incoordination, muscle tremors	Variable	Urine sample
Aujeszky's disease	No	No	Yes	Yes	Respiratory distress, salivation	Pruritus, licking, chewing	None	Signs
Brain abscess	Often	Yes	Yes	Some	Variable	Nystagmus, ataxia, circling, head deviation	Variable	Leucocytosis, suppurative lesion elsewhere
Botulism	No	Yes	No	No	Recumbency later	Incoordination, ataxia, progressive paralysis	No use	Signs
Cerebrocortical necrosis	Yes	Less severe cases	Yes	No	Normal ruminal movements	Muscle tremors, opisthotonus, pupils respond to light, recumbency	Good if early	Age (usually over 6 months), signs, histology, brain fluorescence

Coccidiosis	No	Slight	Yes	No or slight	Diarrhoea/dysentery	Strabismus, tetany, opisthotonus	Poor	Faecal oocyst count
Coenurosis	Unilateral	Yes	Yes	No	Loss of condition	Head deviation, circling, ataxia, head pressing	Surgical – often good	Signs, area
Ergot poisoning	At times	At times	At times	No	Diarrhoea	Drowsiness, convulsions	No therapy	Presence of sclerotia in feed
Fluorosis	No	Yes	No	Some	Dyspnoea, diarrhoea, constipation	Muscular tremor, tetany	Variable	Blood fluorine levels
Furazolidone poisoning (acute)	No	No	Yes	No	Few other signs	Convulsions	Limited value	History of usage
Haemophilus somnus infection	Unilateral	Yes	Yes, later	Yes	Recumbency	Eyes often partly closed, ataxia, convulsions	Variable	Signs, neutropaenia, bacteriology
Hypomagnesaemia	No	No	Yes	Yes	Increased loud heart rate	Opisthotonus, paddling movements	Good if early	Low blood magnesium levels
Infectious bovine rhinotracheitis (nervous)	No	Intermittent	Intermittent	Yes	Anorexia	Incoordination	No therapy	Viral isolation, paired serology
Infectious necrotic hepatitis	No	Yes	Some	Yes	Painful liver, tachypnoea	Hyperaesthesia	Poor	Signs, history, bacteriology
Lead poisoning	Yes	No	Yes	No or slight	Ruminal stasis, diarrhoea	Bellowing, tonic–clonic convulsions, lack of palpebral reflex	Some success	Blood lead levels, liver and kidney post mortem
Lightning strike/ electrocution	Yes	Yes	Yes	No	Paralysis	Paralysis of one or more limbs	Little use	Signs, history
Linseed poisoning	No	Yes acute	Yes	No	Cyanosis, dyspnoea	Opisthotonus, nystagmus	Variable	Linseed feeding

Table 8.18 continued

Disease	*Blindness*	*Dullness*	*Hyperaesthesia*	*Pyrexia*	*Other signs*	*Other nervous signs*	*Response to therapy*	*Diagnosis*
Listeriosis	Often	Yes	No	Yes	Hypopyon, panophthalmitis	Head pressing, circling, head deviation, unilateral facial paralysis	Often poor	Signs
Louping ill	Apparent	No	Yes	Yes	Variable	Jerky stiff movements, incoordination	Variable	Serology
Male fern poisoning	Yes	Yes	No	No	Poor condition	Partial blindness	Variable	History, signs
Malignant catarrhal fever	Yes	Yes	Yes	Yes	Scleral congestion, lymph node enlargement	Muscle tremors, nystagmus, incoordination	Hopeless	Signs
Mannosidosis	No	Slight	Yes	No	Loss of condition	Fine lateral head tremor, vertical head nodding	None	Low tissue α-mannosidase
Meningitis	No	At times	At times	Yes	Anorexia	Opisthotonus, spasm of neck muscles, paddling movements	Good if early	Cerebrospinal fluid cell count
Mercury poisoning	Yes	Yes	No	No	Abdominal pain, diarrhoea	Terminal incoordination, convulsions, recumbency	Variable	Post-mortem kidney mercury levels, history, faeces, urine
Middle ear disease	No	Yes	No	No	Respiratory signs	Head rotation	Often poor	Signs, previous respiratory infection

Nitrate poisoning	No	Yes	No	No	Dyspnoea, diarrhoea, cyanosis	Muscle tremors, staggering gait	Some success if early	Methaemoglobin
Organophosphorus poisoning	No	Yes	No	Yes	Dyspnoea, diarrhoea, salivation, bradycardia	Miosis, muscle tremors, stiff gait	Good	Signs, history
Otitis (non-discharging)	No	Yes	No	No		Head rotation, incoordination	Often poor	Signs, bacteriology
Photosensitization	Some	Some	Some	No	Skin lesions of unpigmented parts exposed to the sun		Good	Signs, history
Progressive ataxia	No	No	No	No	Usually none	Progressive ataxia	None	Signs, breeding, histology
Ragwort poisoning	Yes	Yes	No	Yes	Rectal prolapse, diarrhoea, straining	Frenzy, staggering gait, circling	Usually little value	Signs, history, histology
Selenium poisoning	Yes	Yes chronic	Yes acute	No	Colic, depraved appetite, chronic loss of condition	Head pressing, paralysis	Limited success	Blood and urine levels
Sodium chloride poisoning	Sometimes	Slight	No	No	Excessive thirst, diarrhoea abdominal pain	Paresis, fetlock knuckling	Usually good if early	Serum sodium levels
Sodium monochloroacetate poisoning	No	No	Yes	Variable	Few other signs	Hyperexcitability, aggressiveness, convulsions, paralysis	Little	History, use of herbicide

Table 8.18 continued

Disease	*Blindness*	*Dullness*	*Hyperaesthesia*	*Pyrexia*	*Other signs*	*Other nervous signs*	*Response to therapy*	*Diagnosis*
Spastic paresis	No	No	No	No	Over-straight hock	Abnormal gait	Surgical – good	Signs
Staggers	No	No	Yes	Variable	Profuse salivation	Nystagmus, rocking-horse gait	Good	Signs
Tetanus	No	No	Yes	Yes	Bloat, difficulty in swallowing	Stiff gait, hyperaesthesia, erect ears, raised tail base	Poor	Signs
Urea poisoning	No	No	Yes	Yes	Bloat, dyspnoea	Muscle twitching	Variable	Signs, blood and rumen ammonia levels
Urolithiasis	No	Yes	No	No	Straining		Good if early	Signs
Vitamin A deficiency	Yes	No	No	No	Diarrhoea, bran skin scales	Convulsions, syncope	No use if congenital, good if postnatal	Low plasma and liver levels

From: *Growing Cattle Management and Disease Notes, Part 2 Disease*, A. H. Andrews (1986), published by the Author, Welwyn.

Table 8.19 Differential diagnosis of central nervous problems in adult cattle

Disease	*Blindness*	*Dullness*	*Hyper-aesthesia*	*Pyrexia*	*Other signs*	*Other nervous signs*
Acetonaemia (nervous)	Apparent	Yes	No	No	Constipation, ketone smell	Walking in circles, straddling gait, excessive bellowing
Acidosis	Apparent	Yes	Yes	No	Ruminal stasis, tachycardia	Head deviation, circling, staggering gait, muscle tremors
Aflatoxicosis	Yes	Yes	No	No	Teeth grinding, diarrhoea, jaundice, tenesmus	Walk in circles
Arsenic poisoning	No	Very	Usually no	No	Abdominal pain, fetid diarrhoea	Incoordination, muscle tremors
Aujeszky's disease	No	No	Yes	Yes	Respiratory distress,	Pruritus, licking, chewing
Brain abscess	Often	Yes	Yes	Some	Variable	Nystagmus, ataxia, circling, head deviation
Botulism	No	Yes	No	No	Recumbency later	Incoordination, ataxia, progressive paralysis
Bovine spongiform encephalopathy	Slight	At times	Yes	No	Loss of condition	Progressive ataxia, recumbency, aggression
Cerebrocortical necrosis	Yes	Less severe cases	Yes	No	Normal ruminal movements	Muscle tremors, opisthotonus, pupils respond to light, recumbency

Table 8.19 continued

Disease	*Blindness*	*Dullness*	*Hyper-aesthesia*	*Pyrexia*	*Other signs*	*Other nervous signs*
Coenurosis	Unilateral	Yes	Yes	No	Loss of condition	Head deviation, circling, ataxia, head pressing
Ergot poisoning	At times	At times	At times	No	Diarrhoea	Drowsiness, convulsions
Fluorosis	No	Yes	No	Some	Dyspnoea, diarrhoea, constipation	Muscular tremor, tetany
Furazolidone poisoning (acute)	No	No	Yes	No	Few other signs	Convulsions
Haemophilus somnus infection	Unilateral	Yes	Yes, later	Yes	Recumbency	Eyes often partly closed, ataxia, convulsions
Hypocalcaemia	Apparent	Later	Early	No	Constipation, dilated pupils, no ruminal movements	Excitement early, muscle tremors
Hypomagnesaemia	No	No	Yes	Yes	Increased loud heart rate	Opisthotonus, paddling movements
Infectious necrotic hepatitis	No	Yes	Some	Yes	Painful liver, tachypnoea	Hyperaesthesia
Lead poisoning	Yes	No	Yes	No or slight	Ruminal stasis, diarrhoea	Bellowing, tonic–clonic convulsions, lack of palpebral reflex

Lightning strike/electrocution	Yes	Yes	Yes	No	Paralysis	Paralysis of one or more limbs
Linseed poisoning	No	Yes, acute	Yes	No	Cyanosis, dyspnoea	Opisthotonus, nystagmus
Listeriosis	Often	Yes	No	Yes	Hypopyon, panophthalmitis	Head pressing, head deviation, circling, unilateral facial paralysis
Louping ill	Apparent	No	Yes	Yes	Variable	Jerky, stiff movements, incoordination
Male fern poisoning	Yes	Yes	No	No	Poor condition	Partial blindness
Malignant catarrhal fever	Yes	Yes	Yes	Yes	Scleral congestion, lymph node enlargement	Muscle tremors, nystagmus, incoordination
Mannosidosis	No	Slight	Yes	No	Loss of condition	Fine lateral head tremor, vertical head nodding
Meningitis	No	At times	At times	Yes	Anorexia	Opisthotonus, spasm of neck muscles, paddling movements
Mercury poisoning	Yes	Yes	No	No	Abdominal pain, diarrhoea	Terminal incoordination, convulsions, recumbency
Middle ear disease	No	Yes	No	No	Respiratory signs	Head rotation
Nitrate poisoning	No	Yes	No	No	Dyspnoea, cyanosis, diarrhoea	Muscle tremors, staggering gait

Table 8.19 continued

Disease	*Blindness*	*Dullness*	*Hyper-aesthesia*	*Pyrexia*	*Other signs*	*Other nervous signs*
Organophosphorus poisoning	No	Yes	No	Yes	Dyspnoea, diarrhoea, bradycardia, salivation	Miosis, muscle tremors, stiff gait
Otitis (non-discharging)	No	Yes	No	No		Head rotation, incoordination
Periodic opisthotonus	No	No	Some	No		Periodic spastic attacks
Photosensitization	Some	Some	Some	No	Skin lesions of unpigmented parts exposed to the sun	
Progressive ataxia	No	No	No	No	Muscle weakness, recumbency	Anorexia, rhythmic head movement
Ragwort poisoning	Yes	Yes	No	Yes	Rectal prolapse, diarrhoea, straining	Frenzy, staggering gait, circling
Selenium poisoning	Yes	Yes chronic	Yes acute	No	Colic, depraved appetite, chronic loss of condition	Head pressing, paralysis
Sodium chloride poisoning	At times	Slight	No	No	Excessive thirst, diarrhoea, abdominal pain	Paresis, fetlock knuckling
Sodium monochloroacetate poisoning	No	No	Yes	Variable	Few other signs	Hyperexcitability, aggressiveness, convulsions, paralysis

Spastic paresis	No	No	No	No	Over-straight hock	Abnormal gait
Staggers	No	No	Yes	Variable	Profuse salivation	Nystagmus, rocking-horse gait
Tetanus	No	No	Yes	Yes	Bloat, difficulty in swallowing	Stiff gait, hyperaesthesia, erect ears, raised tail base
Trauma	Yes	Yes	No	No	Unconscious	Unconscious, dilated pupils, poor reflexes
Urea poisoning	No	No	Yes	Yes	Bloat, dyspnoea	Muscle twitching
Urolithiasis	No	Yes	No	No	Straining	

From: *Adult Cattle Management and Disease Notes*, A. H. Andrews (not yet published).

9 Mammary gland

The udder
Mastitis with systemic signs
Mastitis with milk and udder changes
Mastitis with udder changes only
Teats
Some teat lesions

The udder

The udder should be inspected for size, symmetry and abnormal swellings. The surface may show the presence of lesions. In some freshly calved animals there is oedema of the teats, udder and abdominal wall cranial to the udder. Palpation of the udder indicates its consistency, pain, etc., as well as showing areas of induration, abscess formation, etc. The supramammary lymph nodes which are found dorsal to the udder should also be palpated.

Milk should be drawn from the udder and looked at for colour, consistency and smell. Blood in the milk is not uncommon in cows which have recently calved. Proper examination requires the use of a strip cup. Milk samples should be taken for bacteriology. The cellular content of the milk is also of use in indicating inflammation of an acute and chronic nature. Bulk herd cell counts are helpful in indicating subclinical infection.

Indirect methods of showing mastitis involve tests to detect the amount of DNA present due to the number of leucocytes, as is done with the California milk test and Whiteside test. Characteristics of the milk alter with the presence of mastitis and can be assessed. Some other tests have been used such as alteration in conductivity of the milk, but do need further evaluation.

Table 9.1 Some causes of mastitis with systemic signs

Staphylococcus aureus (peracute)
Coliform mastitis (peracute)
Streptococcus dysgalactiae (peracute, acute)
Streptococcus agalactiae (peracute, acute)
Streptococcus uberis (peracute, acute)
Streptococcus zooepidemicus (acute)
Streptococci of Lancefield's Group O (peracute, acute)
Streptococcus pyogenes (peracute, acute)
Streptococcus pneumoniae (peracute)
Escherichia coli (peracute, acute)
Klebsiella pneumoniae (peracute, acute)
Enterobacter aerogenes (peracute, acute)
Actinomyces (Corynebacterium) pyogenes
Pasteurella multocida (peracute)
Pseudomonas aeruginosa (peracute)
Bacillus cereus (peracute)
Candida spp. infection
Saccharomyces spp. infection

Table 9.2 Some causes of mastitis with milk and udder changes

Micrococci (subacute)
Streptococcus zooepidemicus (subacute)
Streptococcus dysgalactiae (acute)
Streptococcus uberis (acute)
Streptococci of Lancefield's Group O (acute)
Staphylococcus epidermidis (subacute)
Staphylococcus aureus (chronic, subacute)
Staphylococcus xylosus
Staphylococcus sciuri
Escherichia coli (acute)
Streptococcus agalactiae (chronic, indurated)
Streptococcus pneumoniae (chronic)
Mycoplasma bovis
Mycoplasma bovigenitalium
Fusiformis necrophorus
Mycobacterium lacticoli
Mycobacterium fortuitum
Candida spp.
Saccharomyces spp.

Table 9.3 Some causes of mastitis with udder changes only

Micrococci
Escherichia coli (chronic)
Staphylococcus aureus (subclinical)
Streptococcus agalactiae (chronic)
Streptococcus dysgalactiae (chronic)
Streptococcus uberis (subclinical)
Streptococcus pneumoniae (chronic)
Streptococcus pyogenes (chronic)

Teats

Besides mastitis, lesions of the teats can be quite common and need to be differentiated (Table 9.4).

History

This can be helpful and does involve knowing whether it is an individual or group problem and the duration of the condition.

Examination

Examination of the lesions is the most important part of diagnosis of teat problems.

Table 9.4 Differential diagnosis of some teat lesions

Blackspot	Black scabby area at teat orifice
Bovine ulcerative mammillitis	Initial oedema then vesicles which rupture leaving ulcers with exudation of serum, then formation of large scabs. Healing takes about 3 weeks. The lesions are painful
Chemical injury (usually teat dips)	Dry, thickened, roughened, discoloured areas around the teat orifice
Chemical injury (concentrated udder wash)	Scab formation over teat end
Chemical injury (chemicals in bedding)	Teat skin irritation of lateral surface
Cowpox	Initial vesicles and pustules usually not seen replaced by 1–2 cm thick, yellow-brown to red scabs
Foot-and-mouth disease	Vesicle formation
Frostbite	Initially pale or red then, if severe, scab at distal end of teat which is lost leaving a red granulation area
Impetigo and folliculitis	Pustule followed by erythema
Insect lesions	Sore areas often denuded of epithelium and with suppuration
Mastitis (peracute)	Oedematous swelling of teat with necrosis and serous exudation
Milking machine damage	Teat duct prolapse. Subcutaneous haemorrhaging
Photosensitization	Oedema and erythema with skin becoming dry and being shed, leaving exudative areas
Pseudocowpox	Local oedema with papule formation. The lesion enlarges and a scab forms. Healing is from centre outwards, producing a ring or horseshoe
Ringworm	Thick encrusted area
Sunburn	Marked reddening and drying of teats with blistering
Teat chaps	Horizontal cracks in teat skin with exudation and scab formation
Teat lacerations	Torn skin which may involve some or all underlying tissues
Teat trauma	Oedema, bruising of teat
Vaccinia infection	Vesicles become pustules and then thick red to brown scabs
Vesicular stomatitis	Vesicles of teat
Warts	Can be elongated and hard white nodules

10 Skin

Abnormalities
Examination
Pruritus
Dermatitis
Alopecia
Pityriasis
Skin nodules
Skin reddening
Scab/crust formation
Skin thickening
Skin conditions in calves and growing cattle
Skin conditions in adult cattle

Skin lesions are common in cattle and can be either primary or secondary. Some are an indication of problems of a generalized nature (see Table 2.8). Most are of parasitic origin. Lesions often involve areas of alopecia and there may be presence or absence of pain and/or pruritus. The lesions themselves may be discrete or diffuse. Discrete ones are vesicles which may rupture to exude serum or lymph; larger ones are known as blebs, bullae or blisters. Other lesions include macules or papules which if larger become nodes or nodules. Pustules can be present containing pus, or other lesions occur with some thickening, oedema or erythema. The area can be covered in exudate which dries to form a scab. In other lesions the skin becomes covered by flakes. If pruritus is intense it can result in removal of the skin surface leading to excoriation and fissures with cracks penetrating into the deeper layers of the skin.

The colour of the skin may alter and show reddening or erythema. In some cases the redness will be intense. In early cases of gangrene the skin will take on a purplish hue and it will feel cold to the touch.

Abnormalities

There can be various abnormalities affecting the sweat glands as well as the structure and appearance of the skin.

Examination

In most cases skin examination should be undertaken following a good general examination to ensure that the lesions are local and not those of a more general problem. Where lesions occur, scraping may be necessary to determine the presence of parasites or fungi. Swabs may be required for assessment of bacteria present. In many cases it will be necessary to take a skin biopsy to determine the cause of the problem.

Pruritus

This is due to irritation of the skin and in many cases is the result of parasitic infestation (Table 10.1). However in some instances it can be more central in origin and originates from the scratch centre. When this occurs it can be due to environmental change as in Aujeszky's disease or it can be functional as in some liver dysfunctions. A few cases of pruritus may occur after the offending stimulus has been lost. This is called 'skin memory'

Table 10.1 Some causes of pruritus

Aujeszky's disease
Chorioptic mange (slight)
Copper deficiency
Ectoparasitic conditions
Eczema
Lice infestation
Mercury poisoning (chronic)
Photosensitization
Psoroptic mange
Pyrexia/pruritus/haemorrhagic syndrome
Sarcoptic mange
Warble fly infestation

and is much more frequently observed in humans and companion animals than cattle.

Dermatitis

This is inflammation of both the epidermal and dermal layers of the skin. There are many causes (Table 10.2).

Table 10.2 Some causes of dermatitis

Allergic
Chemicals
Arsenic
Infections
Bacteria
Dermatophilus congolensis
Fungi
Ringworm
Viruses
Blue tongue
Bovine herpes mammillitis
Bovine malignant catarrh
Cowpox
Foot-and-mouth disease
Mucosal disease
Pseudocowpox
Rinderpest
Vesicular stomatitis
Nutrition
Potatoes
Physical agents
Frostbite
Photosensitization
Sunburn
Trauma

Table 10.3 Some causes of alopecia

Adenohypophyseal hypoplasia
Baldy calves
Chlorinated naphthalene poisoning
Clinical epitheliogenesis imperfecta
Congenital hypotrichosis
Eczema
Familial acantholysis
Folic acid deficiency
Hyperkeratitis
Inherited congenital hypotrichosis
Inherited congenital ichthyosis
Inherited generalized alopecia
Inherited symmetrical alopecia
Iodine deficiency
Lice infestation
Mycotic dermatitis (calves)
Nervous alopecia
Pachyderma
Pyridoxine deficiency
Psoroptic mange
Riboflavin deficiency
Sarcoptic mange
Selenium poisoning (hair at tail base)
Symmetrical alopecia
Thyroid deficiency
Vitamin A deficiency
Zinc deficiency

Table 10.4 Some causes of pityriasis

This is the production of dandruff seen as brown scales on the surface of the skin. It may be caused by:

Chlorinated naphthalenes
Mycotic dermatitis (calves)
Vitamin A deficiency

Table 10.5 Some causes of skin nodules

Acne
Actinobacillosis
Demodex infestation
Lymphomatosis
Mast cell tumours
Melanoma
Papillomatosis
Skin tuberculosis
Sporadic bovine leukosis
Sporotrichosis
Staphylococcus spp. infection
Warble fly infestation

Table 10.6 Some causes of skin reddening

Arsenic poisoning (chronic)
Chorioptic mange
Dermatitis
Eczema
Impetigo (small, localized)
Lice infestation
Midge bites
Parakeratosis
Photosensitization
Ragwort poisoning
Rinderpest
Sarcoptic mange
St John's wort poisoning

Table 10.7 Some causes of skin scab/crust formation

Baldy calves
Bovine viral diarrhoea (chronic)
Chorioptic mange
Dermatitis
Eczema
Lice infestation
Mercury poisoning (chronic around anus, vulva)
Mucosal disease (chronic)
Mycotic dermatitis
Psoroptic mange
Rinderpest
Ringworm
Sarcoptic mange
Zinc deficiency

Table 10.8 Some causes of skin thickening

Angioneurotic oedema
Baldy calves
Cellulitis (tarsal particularly)
Chlorinated naphthalene poisoning
Chorioptic mange
Congenital ichthyosis
Emphysema
Haemorrhage
Hyperkeratosis
Inherited congenital porphyria
Inherited parakeratosis
Lice infestation
Lymphangitis
Midge bites
Milk allergy
Mycotic dermatitis (calves)
Oedema
Pachyderma
Parakeratosis
Photosensitization (oedema)
Psoroptic mange
Sarcoptic mange
Sporadic bovine leukosis
Urticaria (oedema)
Vitamin A deficiency
Zinc deficiency (+ parakeratitis)

Table 10.9 Differential diagnosis of some skin conditions in calves and growing cattle

Disease	*Lesions*
Aujeszky's disease	Marked nervous signs with mutilation of the affected area
Bovine malignant catarrh	Necrosis
Chorioptic mange	Small scabs
Copper deficiency	Depigmentation of hair
Demodectic mange	Nodules and pustules
Ergot poisoning (chronic)	Loss of tissue
Inherited parakeratosis	Parakeratosis
Iodine deficiency	Alopecia
Iodism	Stary coat, much dandruff
Mercury poisoning	Scabby lesions
Molybdenum poisoning	Depigmentation of hair
Mucosal disease	Scabbiness
Mycotic dermatitis	Matting of hair
Papillomatosis	Papillomas
Pediculosis	Self-inflicted lesions
Photosensitization	Reddening, oedema, exudation and sloughing of skin
Psoroptic mange	Papules, scabs
Pyrexia/pruritus/haemorrhagic syndrome	Usually self-inflicted
Ringworm	Thick grey-white encrustations
Sarcocystosis	Loss of hair
Sarcoptic mange	Thickened, wrinkled skin
Vitamin A deficiency	Bran scales
Warble fly	Larvae in subdermal tissue
Zinc deficiency	Parakeratosis

From: *Growing Cattle Management and Diseases Notes, Part 2 Disease,* A. H. Andrews (1986) published by the Author, Welwyn.

Table 10.10 Differential diagnosis of skin conditions in adult cattle

Disease	*Pruritus*	*Alopecia*	*Lesions*	*Main sites*	*Diagnosis*
Aujeszky's disease	Yes	Yes	Marked nervous signs with mutilation of the affected area	Lesion where virus entered	Signs
Bovine malignant catarrh	No	No	Necrosis	Teats, vulva, muzzle, feet skin-horn junction	Signs, necropsy
Chorioptic mange	Yes	No	Small scabs	Base of tail, legs, udder, escutcheon	Skin scraping for parasites
Copper deficiency	No	No	Depigmentation of hair	Body then periorbital area	Plasma copper level, liver copper level
Demodectic mange	Little	Occasionally	Nodules and pustules	Shoulder, forearm, brisket, lower neck	Mites in pus
Ergot poisoning (chronic)	No	No	Loss of tissue	Tips of ears, tail	Presence of ergot in feed
Inherited parakeratosis	No	Yes	Parakeratosis	Limbs, muzzle, underside of jaw	Serum zinc levels
Iodine deficiency	No	Yes	Alopecia	Variable	Low blood protein, blood iodine
Iodism	No	No	Stary coat, much dandruff	Whole body	Use of iodine
Mercury poisoning	Yes	Yes	Scabby lesions	Anus, vulva	Exposure to mercury
Molybdenum poisoning	No	No	Depigmentation of hair	Body, then periorbital area	Plasma copper level

Mucosal disease	No	No	Scabbiness	Body, vulva, scrotum, perineum	Virus isolation, serology
Mycotic dermatitis	No	Yes	Matting of hair	Back, sides of legs, back of udder	Presence of organism
Papillomatosis	No	No	Papillomas	Muzzle, head, neck	Biopsy
Pediculosis	Yes	Yes	Self-inflicted lesions	Shoulders, upper part of neck, head	Lice isolation, presence of eggs
Photosensitization	Yes	No	Reddening, oedema, exudation and sloughing of skin	Unpigmented areas of skin exposed to sun	Signs
Psoroptic mange	Yes	Yes	Papules, scabs	Withers, neck, base of tail	Skin scraping for parasites
Pyrexia/pruritus/ haemorrhagic syndrome	Usually	Yes	Usually self-inflicted	Variable, usually head, neck	Usually on silage
Ringworm	No	Sometimes	Thick grey-white encrustations	Eyes, neck, head, perineum	Hair sample for spore presence
Sarcocystosis	No	Yes	Loss of hair	Variable	Other signs, presence of organism
Sarcoptic mange	Yes	Yes	Thickened, wrinkled skin	Inside thighs, axilla, underside of neck	Skin scraping for parasites
Vitamin A deficiency	No	No	Bran scales	Back, mane	Plasma vitamin A level, liver vitamin A level
Warble fly	Little	No	Larvae in subdermal tissue	Back	Larvae in lesions
Zinc deficiency	No	Yes	Parakeratosis	Limbs, muzzle, vulva	Serum zinc levels

From: *Adult Cattle Management and Disease Notes*, A. H. Andrews (not yet published).

11 Musculoskeletal system

Ataxia
Stiff gait
Staggering gait
Lameness
Myopathy
Arthropathy
Arthritis
Osteodystrophy

The system's main function is to support the body and thereby ensure that the stance and gait of the animal are normal. Diseases of muscles, bones and joints result in locomotory disturbances (e.g. ataxia, Tables 11.1–11.3) and/or changes in posture. Nerves are responsible for functional activity of the muscles and are dealt with under the section on the nervous system (see Chapter 8). Some systemic problems can result in muscular weakness and tremor together with pain and incoordination. Thus it is often necessary to differentiate diseases of the nervous system and other systemic conditions from those of the muscles, skeleton and joints. A common sequel is a varying degree of lameness (Table 11.4).

Table 11.1 Some causes of ataxia

Aujeszky's disease
Botulism
Bovine spongiform encephalopathy
Brain abscess (some cases)
Brain neoplasia (some cases)
Brassica poisoning
Cerebral anoxia (chronic)
Cerebellar disease
Coenurosis
Copper deficiency
Encephalitis
Enzootic bovine leukosis
Familial ataxia
Gid
Haemophilus somnus infection
Hepatitis (some cases)
Hypomagnesaemia
Mannosidosis
Milk allergy
Parturient paresis
Penitrem A poisoning
Photosensitization (severe)
Progressive ataxia
Toxoplasmosis
Water intoxication

Table 11.2 Some causes of stiff gait

Arsenic poisoning
Arthritis
Blackleg
Blue tongue
Calcium deficiency
Cerebrocortical necrosis

Table 11.2 continued

Chlamydial polyarthritis (calves)
Contracted flexor tendons
Copper deficiency
Gas gangrene
Hypertrophic pulmonary osteoarthropathy
Lead poisoning
Louping ill
Malignant oedema
Mercury poisoning (chronic)
Molybdenum poisoning
Mycoplasma bovis infection
Myopathy
Organophosphorus poisoning
Osteomalacia
Parturient paresis
Rickets
Ryegrass staggers
Selenium/vitamin E deficiency
Selenium poisoning (chronic)
Septic arthritis
Spastic syndrome
Strychnine poisoning
Tetanus
Zinc deficiency

Table 11.3 Some causes of staggering gait

Acidosis
Arthropathy
Bovine spongiform encephalopathy
Cereal engorgement
Congestive heart failure (weakness)
Ergot poisoning (acute)
Fat cow syndrome (in calf)
Haemonchosis
Hydrocyanic acid poisoning (subacute)
Hypomagnesaemia
Lead poisoning (acute, subacute)
Lupin poisoning
Mercury poisoning (chronic)
Organophosphorus poisoning
Oxalate poisoning (acute)
Parturient paresis (early)
Penitrem A poisoning
Post-parturient haemoglobinuria
Ragwort poisoning
Rhododendron poisoning
Ryegrass staggers
Transit tetany

Table 11.4 Some causes of lameness

Arthritis
Arthropathy
Blackleg
Blue tongue (laminitis)
Bovine viral diarrhoea (acute)
Brucella abortus (synovitis, bursitis)
Calcium deficiency
Carpal bursitis
Chlamydial polyarthritis
Degenerative joint disease
Digital dermatitis
Dislocations – hip, sacroiliac, stifle, patella, fetlock
Epiphysitis
Erysipelothrix arthritis
Fluorosis (chronic)
Foot-and-mouth disease
Foul in the foot
Fractures – femur, humerus, tibia, radius, pelvis, carpus, tarsus, metacarpal, metatarsal, pedal
Gas gangrene
Haemophilus somnus infection (synovitis)
Hip dysplasia
Inherited arthrogryposis
Inherited multiple ankylosis
Inherited multiple tendon contraction
Inherited osteoarthritis
Joint ill
Laminitis
Leptospirosis (synovitis)
Malignant oedema
Mastitis (staphylococcal)
Mastitis (summer)
Mucosal disease
Muscle injuries – gastrocnemius, hind limb adductor
Mycoplasma bovis infection (arthritis, synovitis)
Myopathy
Myositis
Nerve paralysis – forelimb: suprascapular, brachial, plexus, radial
hindlimb: femoral, obturator, tibial, peroneal, sciatic
Osteochondrosis – stifle, carpus, atlanto-occipital
Osteomalacia
Osteomyelitis
Penetration of sole
Phosphorus deficiency
Rickets
Selenium poisoning
Septic arthritis
Sodium chloride poisoning

Table 11.4 continued

Solar ulceration
Spastic paresis
Streptococcal arthritis (calves)
Subluxation – hip, sacroiliac, stifle, patella, fetlock
Vitamin D deficiency
White line separation
White line sepsis

Muscles

Muscular examination is usually dependent on inspection and palpation. This indicates the general state of the muscles as well as showing any asymmetry between groups. There may also be interference with movement or muscular atrophy. The muscles are usually well rounded in animals in good condition but their borders tend to become more prominent in disease involving wasting.

Bones

Clinical examination again depends on inspection, palpation and checking movement. There may be abnormalities in shape and contour as well as changes in texture and the consistency of bone. Changes can be the result of congenital defects as well as infections, trauma or deficiencies. Radiography is used as an aid to diagnosis but probably not as often as it might be for cattle.

Joints

Palpation, swelling and movement are used in examination. Most problems are the result of inflammation often as a result of trauma or infection. In cases of infected joints problems can often be secondary to a general disease such as septicaemia or pyaemia. Occasionally a severe form of arthritis particularly involving the tarsus is seen in conditions like septic metritis or acute mastitis.

Feet

The feet are often involved in conditions producing lameness. The hoof formation, however, can be a good indicator of insults, nutritional or infectious, as well as being present in some specific disease conditions.

Myopathy

This is a degeneration of the striated skeletal muscle which is non-inflammatory in origin (Table 11.5).

Table 11.5 Some of the causes of myopathy

Inherited
Degenerative myopathy
Muscular hypertrophy
Ischaemia
Due to recumbency, i.e. downer cows
Nutritional
Vitamin E/selenium deficiency (easily most common in cattle)

Table 11.6 Some of the causes of arthropathy

Secondary to
Ageing process
Fluorosis
Joint defects
Nutritional deficiencies
Osteoarthritis
Osteodystrophia fibrosa
Osteomalacia
Phosphorus deficiency
Rapidly growing cattle with limited exercise
Rickets
Traumatic injury

Arthropathy

This is a non-inflammatory change of the articular surfaces of the joints with degeneration and necrosis (Table 11.6). This definition also embraces osteoarthropathy and degenerative joint disease.

Arthritis

This is inflammation of the articular surfaces and synovial membranes of joints. In cattle most cases are the result of infection and may involve just a single joint, particularly if due to local trauma and infection (Table 11.7). Others are congenital, involving several joints. Often they can follow septicaemia or bacteraemia. The condition is very common in calves.

Table 11.7 Some causes of arthritis

Hypogammaglobulinaemia
Local infection
Bacteraemia (navel)
Septicaemia (navel)
Trauma
Bacteria
Actinomyces (Corynebacterium) pyogenes
Brucella abortus
Escherichia coli
Erysipelothrix insidiosa
Fusiformis necrophorus
Haemophilus somnus
Salmonella dublin
Salmonella typhimurium
Staphylococcus spp.
Streptococcus spp.
Mycoplasma
Mycoplasma bovis
Mycoplasma mycoides
Viruses
Bovine viral diarrhoea

Osteodystrophy

This is a failure of normal bone development and is unusual in cattle in developed parts of the world. The main clinical findings involve an enlargement of the bones, distortion of the bones, susceptibility to fracture, lameness or other changes in gait or posture (Table 11.8).

Table 11.8 Some causes of osteodystrophy

Chronic
Solanum malacoxylon poisoning (not UK)
Inherited
Achondroplasia
Chondrodystrophy
Osteogenesis imperfecta
Osteopetrosis
Nutritional
Calcium deficiency
Calcium:phosphorus imbalance
Copper deficiency
Inadequate protein
Phosphorus deficiency
Vitamin A deficiency
Vitamin A toxicity
Vitamin D deficiency
Physiological
Rapid growth

12 Genital system

Male
- External examination

Female
- Vulva
- Vagina
- Rectal examination
- Abortion
- Causes of abortion in heifers and cows

Male

External examination

This initially involves an inspection of the external genitalia from several angles to see if there is asymmetry, abnormal shape, lesions or prepucial discharge. This inspection is best carried out with restraint outside a crush but obviously this does depend on how fractious the animal is.

Scrotal examination

The condition of the scrotum should be assessed and its consistency should be palpated. Again asymmetry should be looked for. The testicles should move freely within the scrotum and any disparity in size noted. Occasionally scrotal herniae occur.

Testicles

The shape and consistency of the testicles require examination. In addition, the epididymis should be felt along its three parts at the caput, corpus and cauda for size and any abnormality. The testicles of dairy breeds are usually larger than those of beef breeds. On average they are 12–16 cm (5–6.5 in) long and 6–8 cm (2–3 in) in diameter. The ductus deferens should also be palpated from the neck of the scrotal sac, proceeding proximally.

Prepuce and penis

The prepucial opening admits two or three fingers. The glans penis can be palpated through the prepucial opening. The glans penis and sigmoid flexure can be palpated through the skin of the prepuce. Cranial to the prepuce is the area where scrotal herniae can be felt.

Rectal palpation

This is of use in examination of the prostate gland, seminal vesicles, ampullae and vas deferens. The hand is placed caudally to detect the pelvic urethra and the vulvourethral muscle. The prostate gland is small and felt as a slight transverse swelling on the cranial part of the pelvic urethra. The paired seminal vesicles can be felt passing cranially and laterally from the cranial end of the pelvic urethra and the neck of the bladder. Their size and shape vary but they are not usually asymmetrical. The ampullae are the dilated terminal ends of the vas deferens and can be felt by pressing the hand between the seminal vesicles and the pelvic floor. The ampullae are softer than the vas deferens. The ductus deferens can be palpated cranial to the ampulla and passes to the inguinal canal.

Penis exposure

A pudendal nerve block can be used to exteriorize the penis. Often the use of sedatives will produce a similar effect. There is however always a slight chance of continued penile exposure and damage. Electroejaculation will also result in extrusion but can cause some distress to the animal. It does, however, allow a semen sample to be taken.

Semen sampling

Besides use of electroejaculation, semen can be collected with an artificial vagina using a cow in oestrus. Details of examination for fertility are beyond the scope of this book but the semen can be examined for presence of bacteria, pus, etc.

Female

Vulva

Any swelling or vulval discharge can be noted. It is then necessary to part the lips and examine the mucosa.

Vagina

Vaginal examination requires a vaginal speculum with a light. It helps in the diagnosis of infections as well as allowing the external cervical os to be inspected.

Rectal examination

This allows the palpation of cervix, uterus and ovaries. Their size, consistency and activity can be assessed. The oviducts are difficult to detect although it is possible in some cases. Problems are normally the cause of infertility and the technique is used for pregnancy diagnosis. These subjects are beyond the scope of this book.

Table 12.1 Some causes of bleeding from the vulva

Anthrax
Bracken poisoning
Injuries
Malicious damage
Parturition
Post-parturient damage
Recent oestrus
Service damage
Uterine rupture
Vaginal tears
Vulval haemorrhage

Table 12.2 Some causes of purulent discharge from the vulva

Corynebacterium (*Actinomyces*) metritis
Cystitis
Endometritis
Granular vaginitis
Infection (local)
Post-parturient metritis
Pustular vulvovaginitis
Pyelonephritis
Pyometra
Tuberculous metritis
Urethritis
Vaginitis
Vulvovaginitis

Abortion

Abortion is often one sign of a group of problems which can also result in stillbirth or the production of weak calves. There are many definitions of abortion but the one favoured by the Ministry of Agriculture for purposes of brucellosis eradication is parturition before 271 days of gestation.

Table 12.3 Some causes of abortion

Actinobacillus spp. infection
Actinomyces (*Corynebacterium*) *pyogenes* infection
Aflatoxicosis
Anthrax
Arsenic poisoning (chronic)
Aspergillus ochraceus poisoning
Bacillary haemoglobinuria
Blue tongue
Bovine viral diarrhoea (acute)
Brucella abortus
Epizootic abortion
Foot-and-mouth disease
Haemophilus somnus infection
Heat stroke (prolonged)
Hyperthermia (prolonged)
Infectious bovine rhinotracheitis
Iodine deficiency
Leptospirosis (acute)
Leptospira hardjo infection
Listerial abortion
Mucosal disease
Mycobacterium avium
Mycoplasma bovigenitalium infection
Mycobacterium bovis (enteric form)
Mycoplasma bovis infection
Mycidia (*Mucor, Absidia* and *Rhizopus* genera)
Penicillium roqueforti infection
Redwater fever
Salmonellosis (acute enteritis)
Sarcosporidiosis
Tick-borne fever
Tuberculosis
Vitamin A deficiency

Table 12.4 Some causes of abortion in heifers and cows and their differentiation

Condition	*Time of abortion*	*Placenta*	*Fetus*
Avian tuberculosis	Any stage	Organism present	—
Bacillary haemoglobinuria	Variable	—	—
Brucellosis	Over 6 months	Cotyledon necrosis, oedematous placenta with leathery plaques. Organism present	Pneumonia in some, organism in fetal stomach
Epizootic abortion	6–8 months	Necrotic cotyledons, brown gelatinous intercotyledonary area	Liver degeneration, ascites, anasarca, oesophageal and tracheal haemorrhages
Foot-and-mouth disease	Variable	—	—
Fungal (*Aspergillus* spp., *Absidia* spp., *Mucor* spp.)	3–7 months	Often yellow areas on cotyledons. Raised yellow leathery intercotyledonary area, organism present	Raised soft skin lesions, organism in fetal stomach
Haemophilus somnus infection	Variable	—	—
Infectious bovine rhinotracheitis	6–8 months	Organism present	Autolysis, organism in fetus
Iodine deficiency	6–9 months	—	Thyroid enlarged
Iodism	6–9 months	Cotyledon necrosis	—
Leptospira hardjo infection	Over 6 months	Oedematous placenta, yellow-brown cotyledons	Organisms in pleural fluid, kidney and liver

Leptospira infections (e.g. *canicola* and *icterohaemorrhagiae*)	Usually over 5 months	—	Organism isolated
Listeriosis	6–9 months	Organism present	No abnormality, organism present in fetal stomach
Mucosal disease	Variable	—	Stunted growth, congenital abnormalities
Q fever	Variable	—	Organism present
Redwater fever	Variable	—	—
Salmonella dublin infection	About 7 months	—	—
Salmonella typhimurium infection	Any time	—	—
Other *Salmonella* spp. infections	Any time	—	—
Sarcocystosis	Variable	—	—
Summer mastitis	Over 5 months	—	Reduced growth
Tickborne fever	7–9 months	—	—
Trichomoniasis	2–4 months	Uterine exudate contains floccules	Macerated fetus, organism in fetal stomach
Tuberculosis	Any stage	Organism present	—
Vibriosis (*Campylobacter fetus* variety *veneralis*)	5–7 months	Semi-opaque petechial haemorrhages, organism present	Pus on peritoneum, organism in fetal stomach
Vitamin A deficiency	Variable	—	Reduced growth

From: *Growing Cattle Management and Disease Notes*, A. H. Andrews (1986) published by the Author, Welwyn.

13 Deaths

Causes of death within 24 hours
Causes of death within 24–48 hours
Causes of death within 48–120 hours

While this book is not concerned with pathology, the speed of death can be some indication of the cause (Tables 13.1–13.3). The position in which the animal has died is also helpful. Thus the animal can have died peacefully resting on its brisket or following convulsive movements on its side with evidence of leg movements.

Table 13.1 Some causes of death within 24 hours

Abomasal ulceration (with severe haemorrhage)
Anaphylaxis (some cases)
Anthrax
Arsenic poisoning (acute)
Aujeszky's disease
Bacillary haemoglobinuria
Blackleg
Bladder rupture (with haemorrhage)
Botulism (peracute)
Carbon tetrachloride poisoning
Cerebral anoxia (acute)
Clostridium perfringens types A, B, C, D, E
Copper deficiency (rare)
Copper poisoning (acute)
Crude oil poisoning
Electrocution
Endocarditis
Enzootic bovine leukosis (a few)
Fluorosis (acute)
Fog fever
Haemonchosis
Haemophilus somnus infection
Haemorrhage (severe)
Heart failure (acute)
Heat stroke
Hemlock poisoning
Hydrocyanic acid poisoning
Hyperthermia
Hypomagnesaemia
Hypothermia
Infectious bovine rhinotracheitis (extensive obstructive bronchiolitis)
Lead poisoning (acute)
Lightning strike
Listeria infection (septicaemia – calves)
Mastitis (coliform – *Enterobacter aerogenes*, *Escherichia coli*)
Mastitis (*Actinomyces* (*Corynebacterium*) *pyogenes*, *Klebsiella pneumoniae*)
Mastitis (peracute staphylococcal)
Mercury poisoning
Myocardial weakness
Nitrate/nitrite poisoning
Organophosphorus poisoning
Parturient paresis
Pasteurellosis (pneumonic)

Table 13.1 continued

Phosphorus poisoning
Ruminal tympany (frothy and gaseous)
Selenium/vitamin E deficiency (peracute)
Shock
Sodium chloride poisoning (acute)
Strychnine poisoning
Thrombosis of vena cava (some cases)
Urea poisoning
Water hemlock poisoning
Yew poisoning

Table 13.2 A few of the causes of death in 24–48 hours

Acidosis (severe)
Arsenic poisoning (subacute)
Aspergillus pneumonia (calf)
Atypical interstitial pneumonia (young cattle)
Aujeszky's disease
Blackleg
Botulism
Bracken poisoning
Cereal engorgement (severe)
Cerebrocortical necrosis
Colisepticaemia (calves)
Copper poisoning (chronic)
Dinitrophenol poisoning
Fascioliasis (acute)
Fog fever
Gas gangrene
Haemophilus somnus infection (acute)
Haemorrhage
Malignant oedema
Mastitis due to *Bacillus cereus*
Mastitis (coliform – *Enterobacter aerogenes, Escherichia coli*)
Mastitis (*Actinomyces* (*Corynebacterium*) *pyogenes, Klebsiella pneumoniae*)
Mastitis (peracute staphylococcal)
Myocardial weakness
Oxalate poisoning (acute)
Parturient paresis
Pasteurellosis
Peritonitis, acute diffuse (with toxaemia)
Pharyngeal phlegmon
Pulmonary oedema (severe)
Ruminal tympany
Salmonellosis (septicaemia – calves)
Selenium poisoning
Selenium/vitamin E deficiency (acute)
Shock
Thrombosis of vena cava (some cases)

Table 13.3 A few of the causes of death in 48–120 hours

Abomasal impaction (if severe)
Abomasal torsion
Abomasal trauma
Acidosis
Arsenic poisoning (subacute)
Aspiration pneumonia
Aujeszky's disease
Blackleg
Bladder rupture
Bovine malignant catarrh (peracute)
Bracken poisoning
Colienteritis (calves)
Colonic torsion
Enterotoxaemia (*E. coli* – calves)
Fog fever
Lead poisoning (subacute)
Leptospirosis (acute)
Listeria infection (meningoencephalitis – calves)
Lungworm infestation
Mastitis
Mucosal disease
Pasteurellosis
Peritonitis, acute diffuse
Salmonellosis

Index

Abomasal dilatation, 79
Abomasitis, 79, 80
Abortion, 198, 199–201
Adult cattle
  congenital neurological disorders in, 158
  diarrhoea in, 88–93
  differential diagnosis of central nervous system
   problems in, 167–171
  differential diagnosis of skin conditions in, 184–185
  respiratory problems in, 129–130
Agalactia, 8
Aggression, causes of, 20
Alanine aminotranferase, measurement of serum levels, 102
Alimentary dilatation, 80
Alimentary system, 59–96
  abomasal dilatation, 79
  abomasitis, 79, 80
  alimentary dilatation, 80
  colic, 95, 96
  constipation, 81, 94, 95
  deglutition, 63, 65
  diarrhoea, 81, 82–93
  enteritis, 80–81
  intestinal obstruction, 79, 80
  mastication, 61
  oesophagus, 65
  peritonitis, 81, 94
  pharyngeal obstruction, 62, 63
  pharyngitis, 61, 63
  pica, 61, 62
  prehension, 60
  regurgitation, 65
  reticulorumen, 66–76
  ruminal atony, 76, 77
  ruminal tympany, 76–79
  salivation, 63, 64
  stomatitis, 61, 62
  tenesmus, 81, 95
Alkaline phosphatase, measurement of serum levels, 102
Allotriophagia, 61, 62
Alopecia, 180

Anaemia, 112–113
Angiocardiogram, 111
Anorexia, *see* Appetite, complete loss
Appetite
  complete loss (anorexia), causes of, 25–26
  reduced, causes of, 24
Art of diagnosis, 1–3
Arthritis, 192–193
Arthropathy, 192
Asthenia, cardiac, 111
Ataxia, 188
Auscultation
  heart, 108–109
  reticulorumen, 72
  thorax, 120–124

Ballotment of reticulorumen, 73
Bedding, 52
Behaviour, 17
Bile pigments, in urine, 136
Bilirubin, measurement of serum levels, 101
Biopsy, liver, 98–99
Bleeding
  from mucous membranes, 48
  from vulva, 198
Blindness, 143
  partial, 143
Bloat, *see under* Reticulorumen: ruminal tympany
Bones, examination of, 191
Breathing, *see* Respiration

Calves
  causes of diarrhoea in, 82–84
  congenital neurological disorders in, 156
  differential diagnosis of central nervous system
   problems in, 159–161
  differential diagnosis of skin conditions in, 182–183
  respiratory problems in, 127–128
  signs of dehydration in, 26

Cardiovascular system, 105–114
  anaemia, 112–113
  heart, 106–111
    abnormal sounds, 109–110
    angiocardiogram, 111
    auscultation, 108–109
    electrocardiogram, 110
    inspection, 107
    palpation, 107
    paracentesis, 111
    percussion, 107
  myocardial weakness or asthenia, 111
  oedema, 113–114
  valvular disease, 111–112
    endocarditis, 112
Catheterization, 133
Cattle movements, 53
Central nervous system problems
  differential diagnosis
    in adult cattle, 167–171
    in calves, 159, 161
    in growing cattle, 162–166
Cerebrospinal fluid examination, 154–155
Circling, causes of, 143–144
Climate, 56
Clinical examination, 5–57
  behaviour, 17
  condition, 14, 15, 17
  conformation, 23
  defaecation, 27
  dehydration, 24, 26–27
  demeanour and temperament, 17–18, 19, 20
  drinking, 24
  eating, 23–24, 25–26
  environment, 50–57
  gait, 20, 22–23
  general appearance, 15–16
  general inspection, 12–48
  history taking, 6–10
  identification, 10–11
  lymph nodes, 48–50
  mucous membranes, 44–48
  nervous system, 141–155
  odours, 48
  posture
    resting, 18, 21
    specific, 18
    standing, 18
  pulse, 40–44
  respiration, 28–34
    depth, 29–31
    dyspnoea, 31, 32–33
Clinical examination, (*cont.*)
  respiration, (*cont.*)
    noises, 34
    respiratory rate, 28–29
    rhythm, 31, 32
    thoracic symmetry, 31
    type, 33–34
  skin, 178
  temperature, 34–40
    fever, 34–40
    hypothermia, 35, 36
    skin, 40
    in toxaemia, 36
  urination, 27
  voice, 23
Colic, 95, 96
Colour
  of mucous membranes, 44–47
  of skin, 181
  of urine, 134
Coma, causes of, 20
Conformation, 23
Congenital neurological disorders
  in adult cattle, 158
  in calves, 156
  in growing cattle, 157
Constipation, 81, 94
Convulsions, causes of, 144–145
Cough, 117–118
Cranial nerves, 148–152
  abductor nerve, 150
  auditory nerve, 150
  facial nerve, 150
  glossopharyngeal nerve, 150–151
  hypoglossal nerve, 152
  oculomotor nerve, 149
  olfactory nerve, 149
  optic nerve, 149
  spinal accessory nerve, 152
  trigeminal nerve, 149–150
  trochlear nerve, 149
  vagus, 151
Cyanosis, causes of, 46

Deaths, 203–206
  within 24–48 hours, 205
  within 24 hours, 204–205
  within 48–120 hours, 206
Defaecation, 27
Deglutition, 63, 65
Dehydration, 24, 26, 27
  causes of, 27
  signs of in calves, 26

Demeanour and temperament, 17–18, 19, 20
  aggression, 21
  coma, 21
  depression, 18, 19
  dullness, 17
  somnolence, 20
Depression
  mild, causes of, 18
  profound, causes of, 19
Dermatitis, 179–180
Diarrhoea, 81, 82–93
  in adult cattle, 88–93
  in calves, 82–84
  in growing cattle, 83–87
Discharge
  mucous membranes, 47–48
  nasal, 116
  vulval, 198
Disinfection procedures, 52–53
Drainage, 53
Drinking, 24
Dullness, mild, causes of, 17
Dyspnoea, 31
  causes of, 32–33

Eating, 23–24, 25–26
Electrocardiogram, 110
Electroencephalography, 155
Emaciation, causes of, 16
Emphysema, 123
  pulmonary, 126, 127
Endocarditis, 112
Endoscopic examination, thorax, 124
Enteritis, 80–81
Environment, 50–57
  indoors, 51–54
    bedding, 52
    cattle movements, 53
    disinfection procedures, 52–53
    drainage, 53
    flooring, 53
    light, 53
    method of feeding, 53–54
    other buildings, 53
    reproduction management, 54
    space allowances, 52
    ventilation, 52
  outdoors, 54–57
    climate, 56
    feed supplements, 57
    fertilizer usage, 56
    grassland management, 55–56
    plant types, 56

Environment, (*cont.*)
  outdoors, (*cont.*)
    position, 54–55
    shelter, 56
    soil type, 55
    stocking level, 55
    water supply, 57

Faecal examination, 76
Feeding
  method of, 53–54
  supplements, 57
Feet, examination of, 191
Fertilizer usage, 56
Fever, 35–40
  fluctuation, causes of, 39
  mild, causes of, 37
  moderately severe, causes of, 38
  severe, causes of, 39
Flocculation tests, 101–102
Flooring, 53

Gait
  clinical examination of, 20, 22–23
  staggering, 189
  stiff, 188–189
Gammaglutamyltransferase, measurement of serum levels, 102
General appearance of animals, 15–16
General condition of animals, 15, 16, 17
General inspection of animals, 12–48
Genital system, 195–201
  female
    abortion, 198–201
    rectal examination, 197–198
    vagina, 197
    vulva, 197, 198
  male
    external examination, 196–197
    penis exposure, 197
    prepuce and penis, 196
    rectal palpation, 196–197
    scrotum, 196
    semen sampling, 197
    testicles, 196
Glucose, in urine, 136
Glutamate dehydrogenase, measurement of serum levels, 102
Grassland management, 55–56
Growing cattle
  congenital neurological disorders in, 157
  diarrhoea in, 83–87

Growing cattle, (*cont.*)
  differential diagnosis of central nervous system problems in, 162–166
  differential diagnosis of skin conditions in, 182–183
  respiratory problems in, 128–129

Haematuria, 134
Haemoglobinuria, 135
Hair, rough, causes of, 16
Head carriage, causes of alteration in, 142
Heart, 106
  examination of, 106–111
    angiocardiogram, 111
    auscultation, 108–109
    electrocardiogram, 110
    inspection, 107
    palpation, 107
    paracentesis, 111
    percussion, 107
  sounds
    abnormal, 109–110
    character, 108
    frequency, 109
    rhythm, 108
    volume, 108
Hepatitis, 103, 104
History-taking, 6–10
  nervous system problems, 141–2
Hyperaemia of skin, 181
Hypothermia, 35, 36

Identification of animals, 10–11
Inappetite, *see* Appetite, reduced
Incoordination, causes of, 145
Intestinal obstruction, 79, 80

Jaundice, 100–101
  causes of, 46
Joints, examination of, 191

Ketones, in urine, 136

Laboured respiration, 31, 32–33
Lactic dehydrogenase, measurement of serum levels, 102
Lameness, 190
Laparotomy
  liver, 103
  reticulorumen, 75
Laryngitis, 125
Larynx, 118
Light, 53
Liver, 97–104
  biopsy, 98–99
  external palpation, 98
  hepatitis, 103, 104
  jaundice, 100–109
  laboratory testing, 99–100
  liver function tests, 101–104
    alanine aminotransferase, 102
    alkaline phosphatase, 102
    exploratory laparotomy, 103
    flocculation tests, 101–102
    gamma glutamyltransferase, 102
    glutamate dehydrogenase, 102
    lactic dehydrogenase, 102
    paracentesis, 103–104
    proprionate conversion test, 103
    serum bilirubin, 101
    sorbitol dehydrogenase, 102
    sulphobromophthalein test, 101
    ultrasound, 103
Lymph nodes
  examination of, 48–50
    prefemoral (precrural), 50
    prescapular, 50
    submandibular or submaxillary, 49
    superficial inguinal, 50
    supramammary, 50
    suprapharyngeal (retropharyngeal), 50

Mammary gland, 173–176
  mastitis, 174–175
  teats, 175–176
  udder, 174
Mastication, 61
Mastitis
  with milk and udder changes, 175
  with systematic signs, 174
  with udder changes only, 175
Metal detection, 76
Micturition, 27
  frequent, 132
Milk yield
  causes of fall in
    gradual, 9
    sudden, 8
Mouth lesions, causes of, 60
Mucous membranes
  examination of, 44–48
    colour, 44–47
    discharge, 47–48
    heamorrhages, 48
    swelling, 48
Muscles, examination of, 191

Muscle tremor, causes of, 146
Muscular rigidity, causes of, 145
Musculoskeletal system, 187–194
  arthritis, 192–193
  arthropathy, 192
  ataxia, 188
  bones, 191
  feet, 191
  joints, 191
  lameness, 190
  muscles, 191
  myopathy, 191–192
  osteodystrophy, 193–194
  staggering gait, 189
  stiff gait, 188–189
Myoglobinuria, 135
Myopathy, 191–192

Nasal cavities and sinuses, 117
Nasal discharge, 116
Nephrosis, 136–137
Nervous system, 139–171
  alteration in head carriage, 142
  blindness, 143
    partial, 143
  cerebrospinal fluid examination, 154–155
  circling, 143–144
  clinical signs, 140–141
  congenital neurological disorders
    in adult cattle, 158
    in calves, 156
    in growing cattle, 157
  convulsions, 144–145
  cranial nerves, 148–152
    abductor nerve, 150
    auditory nerve, 150
    facial nerve, 150
    glossopharyngeal nerve, 150–151
    hypoglossal nerve, 152
    oculomotor nerve, 149
    olfactory nerve, 149
    optic nerve, 149
    spinal accessory nerve, 152
    trigeminal nerve, 149–150
    trochlear nerve, 149
    vagus, 151
  differential diagnosis of central nervous system problems
    in adult cattle, 167–171
    in calves, 159–161
    in growing cattle, 162–166
  dilated pupils, 148
  history taking, 141–142
Nervous system, (*cont.*)
  incoordination, 145
  muscle tremor, 146
  muscular rigidity, 145
  nystagmus, 146–147
  ophthalmoscopic examination, 154
  opisthotonus, 147
  paralysis, 147–148
  peripheral nerves, 152
  sluggish pupillary reflex, 148
  spinal examination, 154
  spinal reflexes, 152–154
    deep, 154
    in diagnosis of neurological disorders, 153
    organic, 154
    superficial, 152, 154
Nystagmus, causes of, 146–147

Odours, 48
Oedema, 113–114
Oesophagus, 65
Ophthalmoscopic examination, 154
Opisthotonus, causes of, 147
Osteodystrophy, 193–194

Palpation
  heart, 107
  liver, 98
  rectal, 196–197
  reticulorumen, 71
  thorax, 119
Paracentesis
  heart, 111
  liver, 103–104
  reticulorumen, 75
Paralysis, causes of, 147–148
Penis, examination of, 196, 197
Percussion
  heart, 107
  reticulorumen, 71–72
  thorax, 119–120
Peripheral nerve examination, 152
Peritonitis, 81, 94
pH, of urine, 135
Pharyngeal obstruction, 62, 63
Pharyngeal paralysis, causes of, 65
Pharyngitis, 61, 63
Pica, 61, 62
Pityriasis, 180
Plant types, 56
Pneumonia, 125–126
Polydipsia, 133
Polyuria, 132

Poor condition, causes of, 15
Poor growth, causes of, 14
Posture
  resting, 18, 21, 22
  specific, 18
  standing, 18
Prehension, 60
Prepuce and penis, examination of, 196, 197
Proprionate conversion test, 103
Protein, in urine, 135–136
Pruritus, 178–179
Pulmonary congestion, 126, 127
Pulmonary emphysema, 126, 127
Pulse, 40–44
  amplitude, 43–44
  rate, 40–43
  rhythm, 43
Pupillary reflex, sluggish, causes of, 148
Pupils, dilated, causes of, 148
Pyrexia, *see* Fever

Radiography, thorax, 124
Râles fluid, 122–123
Rectal examination, 73–75
  genital system, 196, 197–198
  urinary system, 133
Recumbency, causes of, 22
Reddening of skin, 181
Regurgitation, 65
Reluctance to move, causes of, 23
Renal function tests, 136
Reproduction, management of, 54
Respiration, 28–34
  depth, 29–31
  dyspnoea, 31, 32–33
  laboured, 31, 32–33
  noises, 34
  respiratory rate, 28–29
  rhythm, 31, 32
  thoracic symmetry, 31
  type, 33–34
Respiratory system, 115–130
  cough, 117–118
  diagnosis of problems
    in adult cattle, 129–130
    in calves, 127–128
    in growing cattle, 128–129
  examination of thorax, 118–124
    auscultation, 120–124
    endoscopic examination, 124
    palpation, 119
    percussion, 119–120
Respiratory system, (*cont.*)
  examination of thorax, (*cont.*)
    radiography, 124
    thoracocentesis, 124
  laryngitis, 125
  larynx and trachea, 118
  nasal cavities and sinuses, 116–117
  nasal discharge, 116
  pneumonia, 125–126
  pulmonary congestion, 126
  pulmonary emphysema, 126, 127
  rhinitis, 125
  tracheitis bronchitis, 125
Reticulorumen, 66–76
  abdominal size reduction, 71
  auscultation, 72
  ballotment, 73
  combined ausculatation and percussion, 72
  exploratory laparotomy, 75
  external palpation, 71
  faecal examination, 76
  inspection, 67, 70–71
  metal detection, 76
  normal ruminal cycle, 67, 68
  paracentesis, 75
  percussion, 71–72
  rectal examination, 73–75
  ruminal atony, 76, 77
  ruminal fluid examination, 76
  ruminal movements
    absent, 69
    depressed, 69
    increased, 68
  ruminal tympany, 76–79
    primary, 78
    secondary, 78–79
Rhinitis, 125
Ruminal atony, 76, 77
Ruminal fluid examination, 76
Ruminal movements
  absent, 69
  depressed, 69
  increased, 68
Ruminal tympany, 76–79
  primary, 78
  secondary, 78–79
Rumination cycle, 68

Salivation, increased, 63, 64
Scab/crust formation, 181
Scrotum, examination of, 196
Semen sampling, 197
Shelter, 56

Skin, 177–185
  abnormalities, 178
  alopecia, 180
  dermatitis, 179–180
  differential diagnosis of skin conditions
    in adult cattle, 184–185
    in calves and growing cattle, 182–183
  examination, 178
  nodules, 181
  pityriasis, 180
  pruritus, 178–179
  reddening, 181
  scab/crust formation, 181
  thickening, 182
Sleepiness, causes of, 19
Snoring, causes of, 34
Soil type, 55
Somnolence, causes of, 19
Sorbitol dehydrogenase, measurement of serum levels, 102
Space allowances, 52
Specific gravity, of urine, 135
Spinal examination, 154
Spinal reflexes, 152–154
  deep, 154
  in diagnosis of neurological disorders, 153
  organic, 154
  superficial, 152, 154
Staggering gait, 189
Stertor, causes of, 34
Stiff gait, 188–189
Stocking level, 55
Stomatitis, 61, 62
Straining, 81, 95
Sulphobromophthalein test, 101
Swallowing, 63, 65

Teats, 175–176
Temperature, 34–40
  fever, 34–40
    fluctuation, 39
    mild, 37
    moderately severe, 38
    severe, 39
  hypothermia, 35, 36
  skin, 40
  in toxaemia, 36
Tenesmus, 81, 95
Testicles, examination of, 196
Thorax, examination of, 118–124
  auscultation, 120–124
    bronchial lung sounds, 121
    dry rales, 122
Thorax, (*cont.*)
  auscultation, (*cont.*)
    dullness, 121
    emphysema, 123
    fluid rales, 123
    pleuritic rub, 123–124
    vesicular murmur, 121
  endoscopic examination, 124
  palpation, 118–119
  percussion, 119–120
  radiography, 124
  thoracocentesis, 124
Toxaemia, causes of, 36
Trachea, 118
Tracheitis bronchitis, 125

Udder, 174
Ultrasound examination, liver, 103
Urinalysis, 133–136
  bile pigments, 136
  colour, 134
  deposits, 136
  glucose, 136
  haematuria, 134
  haemoglobinuria, 135
  ketones, 136
  myoglobinuria, 135
  odour, 134
  pH, 135
  protein, 135–136
  quantity, 134
  specific gravity, 135
  transparency, 134
Urinary system, 131–137
  catheterization, 133
  frequent micturition, 132
  nephrosis, 136–137
  polydipsia, 133
  polyuria, 132
  rectal examination, 133
  urinalysis, 133–136
Urination, 27

Vagina, examination of, 197
Ventilation, 52
Voice, 23
Vomiting, causes of, 70
Vulva
  bleeding or discharge from, 198
  examination of, 197

Water supply, 57
Weakness, causes of, 21